Child and Adolescent Mental Health Services

An Operational Handbook

Edited by

Greg Richardson & Ian Partridge

Gaskell

For Dr Tom Pitt-Aikens
– who understood the importance
of 'the good authority'

Cover picture courtesy of Getty Images/© Dick Makin

Chapter 25 is a revised version of material originally published in *Child Psychology and Psychiatry Review*, © Blackwell Publishing Ltd

Gaskell is an imprint of the Royal College of Psychiatrists,
17 Belgrave Square, London SW1X 8PG
http://www.rcpsych.ac.uk

British Library Cataloguing-in-Publication Data
A catalogue record for this book is available from the British Library.
ISBN 1-901242-96-X

Distributed in North America by Balogh International Inc.

Printed in Great Britain by Bell & Bain Limited, Glasgow, UK

Contents

List of contributors   vii

Acknowledgements   ix

1   Introduction   1
     Ian Partridge and Greg Richardson

2   CAMHS in context   7
     Greg Richardson

3   Structure, organisation and management of CAMHS   16
     Ian Partridge, Nick Jones and Greg Richardson

4   Clinical governance   21
     Greg Richardson

5   CAMHS and the law: the Children Act, the Mental Health   27
     Act, child protection, consent and confidentiality
     Caroline Harris, Ian Partridge and Greg Richardson

6   Multi-disciplinary working   38
     Ian Partridge, Greg Richardson, Geraldine Casswell and Nick Jones

7   Evidence-based practice   46
     Juliette Kennedy and Ian Partridge

8   User participation – participatory appraisal   55
     Caroline Keir, Janet Harris and Barbara Webb

9   Training   61
     Nick Jones, Ian Partridge and Barry Wright

10   Court work   66
     Greg Richardson and Geraldine Casswell

11   Strategies for moving into Tier 1   75
     Greg Richardson and Ian Partridge

12   Liaison and consultation with Tier 1 professionals   82
     Greg Richardson and Ian Partridge

13   Referral management   91
     Sophie Roberts and Ian Partridge

14 Structuring and managing treatment options   96
   Ian Partridge, Geraldine Casswell, Nick Jones, Greg Richardson
   and Barry Wright

15 Paediatric liaison   107
   Christine Williams and Barry Wright

16 Day patient services   112
   Rosie Beer

17 In-patient psychiatric care   117
   Greg Richardson, Geraldine Casswell, Nick Jones and Ian Partridge

18 Deliberate self-harm   126
   Barry Wright and Greg Richardson

19 Learning disabilities services   131
   Christine Williams and Barry Wright

20 Autistic spectrum disorders services   142
   Christine Williams and Barry Wright

21 Attentional problems services   150
   Barry Wright and Christine Williams

22 Eating disorders services   157
   Ian Partridge and Greg Richardson

23 Bereavement services   161
   Barry Wright and Ian Partridge

24 Drug and alcohol teams   167
   Norman Malcolm

25 Parenting risk assessment service   174
   Ian Partridge, Geraldine Casswell and Greg Richardson

26 Forensic services   178
   Sue Bailey

27 Neuropsychology and neuropsychiatry services   185
   Helen Prescott and Ian Partridge

   Glossary   189

   References   192

   Index   209

Contributors

Sue Bailey OBE, Consultant Adolescent Forensic Psychiatrist, Adolescent Forensic Services, Bolton, Salford and Trafford Mental Health Partnership

Rosie Beer, Consultant Child and Adolescent Psychiatrist, Little Woodhouse Hall, 18 Clarendon Road, Leeds LS2 9NT

Geraldine Casswell, Consultant Clinical Psychologist, York

Caroline Harris, Clinical Psychologist, Children's Centre, 24 Brompton Road, Northallerton DL6 1EA

Janet Harris, Academic director, Health Sciences, Continuing Professional Development Centre, University of Oxford

Nick Jones, Service Manager, Limetrees Child Adolescent & Family Unit, 31 Shipton Road, York YO30 5RE

Caroline Keir, West Yorkshire Strategic Health Authority, Blenheim House, Duncombe Street, West One, Leeds LS1 4PL

Juliette Kennedy, Specialist Registrar in Child and Adolescent Psychiatry, North Yorkshire Specialist Registrar Training Scheme, The Deanery, University of Leeds

Norman Malcolm, Consultant Child and Adolescent Psychiatrist, Child and Adolescent Service, Fieldhead Buisiness Centre, 2–8 St Martin's Avenue, Listerhills, Bradford BD7 1LG

Ian Partridge, Social Worker, Formerly at Lime Trees, York

Helen Prescott, Consultant Clinical Psychologist, South Child and Adolescent Mental Health Team, and Academic Unit of Child and Adolescent Mental Health, 12A Clarendon Road, Leeds LS2 9NN

Greg Richardson, Consultant Child and Adolescent Psychiatrist, Lime Trees Child Adolescent & Family Unit, 31 Shipton Road, York YO30 5RE

Sophie Roberts, Specialist Registrar in Child and Adolescent Psychiatry, Yorkshire Regional Training Scheme

Barbara Webb, Social Science Researcher in Health Evaluation Studies, York

Christine Williams, Consultant Clinical Psychologist, Limetrees Child Adolescent & Family Unit, 31 Shipton Road, York YO30 5RE

Barry Wright, Consultant Child and Adolescent Psychiatrist, Limetrees Child Adolescent & Family Unit, 31 Shipton Road, York YO30 5RE

Acknowledgements

The editors wish to thank the authors for their contributions and for keeping to deadlines with good humour while continuing to provide a clinical service in their busy posts; all our colleagues, secretarial, community and in-patient, at Lime Trees in York for putting the ideas of this book into practice; all colleagues, past and present, from whose ideas, insights and practice we have learnt, borrowed and at times downright stolen; the families with whom we have worked and from whom we have been informed in the development of both clinical practice and service provision; and finally, our own families.

CHAPTER 1

Introduction

Ian Partridge and Greg Richardson

'The world is disgracefully managed, one hardly knows whom
to complain to.'
Ronald Firbank, Vainglory

Purpose and scope of the book

Child and adolescent mental health services (CAMHS) comprise a
small, unusual speciality that is often ill understood by those who
work within, and those trying to use, them. In an attempt to make
order out of chaos, *Together We Stand* (NHS Health Advisory Service,
1995a) offered a review of, and a strategic framework for, the organisation and management of CAMHS. This strategic approach was
sanctioned by the House of Commons Health Committee (1997) and
provided the benchmarks against which CAMHS have been measured
(Audit Commission, 1999). The present handbook describes how the
theory and strategic framework described in *Together We Stand* can be put
into practice by applying principles of clinical management to the
delivery of CAMHS. This is not a clinical text, although the provision of
any service must be thoroughly informed by a relevant understanding of
clinical need and practice, but is rather a description of how the nuts
and bolts of a CAMHS can be put together to provide a robust, patient-
centred, clinically effective service.

The handbook is therefore geared to those from all disciplines
working in CAMHS as well as those responsible for their organisation.
The editors also consider that the handbook will be helpful to
commissioners, as it details how services should be organised to ensure
value for money when commissioning CAMHS at whatever level (Morley
& Wilson, 2001). The text is underpinned by research evidence as well
as government policy but also by reference to experience, achievement
and opinion.

The handbook addresses the interface between all tiers and the
development of effective operational structures that allow for professional functioning in an integrated fashion. It is not a textbook
describing clinical work at any one tier, but describes the organisation
of CAMHS delivery at each of the tiers. It is not a textbook for Tier 1

professionals looking to develop services for children with mental health problems. However, the importance of the support of Tier 1 and the interface between Tier 1 and other CAMHS provision is emphasised in the two chapters (10 and 11) devoted to that topic. The development of formal links as well as informal understanding of relative functions is part of the relationship building that is at the core of the effective operation of CAMHS.

The developing role of the voluntary sector and client interest/support/pressure groups has affected the nature of service provision. Links must be developed and effective networks established with such groups so that they can truly become partners in service delivery. The voluntary sector has developed differently in different parts of the country, with different agencies taking different priorities. It is therefore difficult to be prescriptive. However, voluntary agencies must be involved in the planning and development of CAMHS.

The incorporation of users' views is an integral part of working in CAMHS, as work is impossible without therapeutic alliances. Users' and carers' perspectives on services should also be the subject of frequent audit.

Principles considered

The overarching principles considered in the handbook that underpin CAMHS delivery are discussed under separate headings below.

Multi-agency, multi-professional liaison, cooperation and management

Children come into daily contact with any number of different professionals who influence their mental health. Any agency that purports to be interested in the mental health of children must work with all those professionals, whatever agency, voluntary or statutory, or profession they come from. CAMHS must therefore work with all other agencies involved with children. Similarly, a competent CAMHS cannot hope to meet children's needs without the input of different disciplines, each offering differing perspectives and knowledge bases. Professional boundaries, which encourage professional imperialism, have no place in a service that puts children and their families at its centre.

Systemic approaches

Children thrive in some systems and do badly in others (Rutter *et al*, 1979). An individual needs assessment, looking at each child, does not always serve them well, and can often lead to stigmatisation and foster low self-esteem. This handbook has therefore taken a systemic approach, and looks at organisational matters that promote mental health rather than individual interventions with individual children. This does not mean that children with individual problems such as autism or anorexia nervosa do not require management packages tailored to their needs, but those packages must be provided in a manner and within an organisational structure that systemically support their mental health. For example, an organisation that provides support and therapy to a family whose daughter has anorexia nervosa is likely to be more successful than one that concentrates on the child. This handbook is based on the premise that a systemically healthy CAMHS will be more effective than a collection of non-interacting mental health professionals.

Clear structure, terms of reference and operational policy

In order to meet a fluctuating, but generally increasing, demand upon services, the organisational structure of any CAMHS must be explicit in terms of both the service that can be offered and the service that cannot. This will involve a degree of prioritisation and, at times, rationing. This position is often muddied by the creation of waiting lists in acceptance of the out-of-date mechanics of responding to referrals rather than managing and restructuring the referral process. CAMHS need to move away from the linear notion of referrals, which is clearly inadequate as only 10% of children with mental disorders and mental health problems are referred to such a service. A system is required that involves work with children and families based upon need, through multi-agency and multi-professional liaison, cooperation and management.

Integration between tiers

The advantage of such organisation is to move away from a system based upon finished consultant episodes and face-to-face contacts, with the consequent medicalisation of child and family development, to a system where intensity of input is geared to complexity of need. The tiered system is one of organisational structure rather than of clinical hierarchy, each CAMHS professional having the potential to work at, or with, more than one tier. Different services will have both different resource levels and different skill mixes, and this will affect their provision. A CAMHS will need to have sufficient professionals within it to provide a comprehensive Tier 2 service, or to form a comprehensive range of Tier 3 teams. However, each of the identified clinical needs can be managed at different positions within the tiered system, depending upon local circumstances. The effective management of CAMHS is dependent on recognition of the interface between the tiers, and a close working integration of them all. In clinical terms, a linear approach to the tiered system will result in its failure, whereas a systemic understanding will allow it to function effectively.

Integration of organisational structure

While CAMHS are generally small, they are sufficiently different from other health service provision that they require their own discrete managerial and organisational structure. Only then will there be allowance for the greater sophistication and specificity in understanding of service delivery and consequent financial management, including effective costing, of the different aspects of service provision. An example of the need for an understanding of CAMHS complexity and the integration of all tiers is in the commissioning and provision of Tier 4 in-patient services. The need for such services may decline with effective community provision at Tiers 1, 2 and 3, but they will still be required, albeit possibly with fewer beds. In the short term, such services may appear both over-expensive and over-staffed, thereby offering the scope for financial savings in times of cutbacks. However, if locality CAMHS withdraw resources from Tier 4 provision, such provision will disappear and not be there on the few occasions when it is required. Such a position of disintegrated tiers is short-sighted, for when Tier 4 is required it will no longer be available and young people will be placed in a service a long way from home, with which their carers are unfamiliar and which is likely to be very expensive. The integration of the tiers rather than fragmentation of CAMHS will allow for a full provision of services for young people from their communities, through to the most specialist provision.

Caring for the carers

A service that does not care for itself is likely to have difficulty caring for others – a fact often overlooked within the caring professions. Working in CAMHS is a tiring and often emotionally draining experience. There must be formal lines of responsibility, accountability and supervision in place, as well as access to training, so that people feel professionally secure and supported by the organisation and their colleagues. A sense of perspective must be maintained so that we do not take ourselves too seriously. There is a place for insensitivity, black humour, prejudice, irritation, frustration and irrationality – all those defence mechanisms essential to our sanity. There is a myth of the objective, detached professional who can shed personality, beliefs and values on entering a professional arena – it is a myth that can lead to burn-out and professional under-functioning. CAMHS work with reality rather than ideals. A simple structural entity can aid this process, namely the staff room or common room. This should be a place wherein the shackles of professional responsibility can be loosened in the comfy cushion of shared lunch or shared coffee, a place where folk can meet rather than professionals assemble.

Evidence-based practice

The Children Act 1989 requires that any intervention into a child or family's life should result in a demonstrably better situation for the child than not intervening. This is a principle, along with the Hippocratic injunction of 'first, do no harm', that can and should inform our clinical practice. In CAMHS we are faced with a wide range of what can broadly be termed 'mental health issues'; we face a very small range of specific diagnosable mental illnesses (Meltzer *et al*, 2000), although public perspectives of referral to a CAMHS will tend to focus upon the latter. Any service provision for members of society cannot be an exact science, ratified by double-blind, randomly controlled trials: the care, support and treatment offered is as much an art as a science. Just as clinical practice will develop in the light of experience, so will organisational structures. Referral to a CAMHS may result in the labelling and stigmatisation of the child and family, as well as in the de-skilling of the parent.

A systemic understanding must always inform our knowledge of the evidence base. Our work should, of course, be focused, problem solving, collaborative and, where possible, short term. Beyond this we should always consider the effect of any CAMHS intervention, which starts in the mind of the child and family long before their first consultation with the referrer. When considering a CAMHS response, those processes preceding referral must be weighed in the balance of mental health pros and cons, so that the response is geared to positive mental health rather than increasing mental health problems.

Services described

Throughout this book the above principles are paramount and guide the service delivery described. To avoid repetition, the following principles can be considered to guide the authors of all the chapters in both the management of the service and the development of effective clinical provision:

- The CAMHS is based on multi-disciplinary working.
- It represents a responsive service that offers advice and support, and that avoids stigmatisation and the disempowering of families, that is, a service that is child and family centred and that dovetails with services from other agencies.

- The CAMHS takes on board the social, educational, emotional and medical needs of the young person and family.
- The service provides clear information to other services and agencies about routes of referral and consultation.
- There is a clear operational policy for each professional, team and service that details skills, accessibility and comprehensiveness.

This handbook was conceived as a manual for those wishing to put their CAMHS in order. Inevitably it takes a CAMHS perspective. However, the need for CAMHS to work with other agencies and for them to understand CAMHS is overwhelming and the principles underlying the handbook dictate a multi-agency perspective.

The services described in this book are based within the legislative framework of England, much of which also pertains to Scotland, Northern Ireland and Wales. There will be differences in details, as a result of initiatives in the devolved United Kingdom (e.g. National Assembly for Wales, 2001). However, the principles of CAMHS delivery will remain the same if services are based on need and effectiveness rather than professional or legal nicety.

Any service exists, as indeed do patients/clients, in a context and, as such, both influence and are influenced by relational factors, be they internal (within a CAMHS) or external (e.g. government or trust policy). Organisational change within the National Health Service has no discernible end-point, so this handbook is heavily informed by reference to 'what works' for both provider and recipient of CAMHS provision, but will clearly have to develop as government policies, societal mores and research dictates.

Some terms used in child and adolescent mental health are confusing. There is therefore a glossary of problematic terms at the end of the handbook to define terms used within the handbook. Throughout the book the term 'service' will apply to a CAMHS, while the term 'team' will be applied to Tier 3 teams working within CAMHS or across agencies.

CHAPTER 2

CAMHS in context

Greg Richardson

'Maps for the future can be drawn only by those who have deeply studied the past.'
Camille Paglia, *Sexual Personage*

Introduction

Over the years, child and adolescent mental health services (CAMHS) have had disparate homes. Local-authority-based child guidance clinics and health-service-based in-patient units only really came together in 1974. At that time there was a recognition that mental health services for children and adolescents should be based in the community rather than in institutions (Department of Health and Social Security, 1975). Now that they are based in health services, the idea and functioning of multi-disciplinary services and teams can represent a mystery to doctor-led, referral-based health systems. As a result, CAMHS have often been prey to neglect and idiosyncratic clinical practice, often of an out-standing nature. However, in the early 1990s a number of factors led to the greater scrutiny of the organisation and functioning of this small, peculiar part of the health service.

Problems in the management of CAMHS

Media response to children's behaviour

The behaviour of our children and teenagers has often provided a barometer for public perceptions of the stability or otherwise of the social order of the day (Pearson, 1983). During the 1980s and 1990s, there arose a greater media focus upon the activities of young people, declining family values and declining notions of parental and individual responsibility. Moral panic regarding rises in single parenthood, teenage pregnancies and divorces rates, as well as sensational events such as the murder of Jamie Bulger by young children, moved the question of children's behaviour and psychology to the centre of social and political debate.

Child abuse

There was a growing public acknowledgment of the abuse of children but there also developed an obsession with the idea of children being torn from their innocent parents. Professionals working with children were in danger of the double-bind alternatives of being perceived as doing too little or of being indiscriminate zealots espying abuse in the most innocent of parent–child interactions. Documents such as the *Report of the Inquiry into Child Abuse in Cleveland* (Butler-Sloss, 1987) called attention to the need for agencies to work together, which was not a new concept but was one that had found its time.

The need for inter-agency collaboration

Publications in the field of social services, such as *Children in the Public Care* (Department of Health & Social Services Inspectorate, 1991), a precursor of *Quality Protects* (Department of Health, 1999b), education, such as the Audit Commission's *Getting in on the Act* (Audit Commission, 1992), and health, such as *With Health in Mind* (Kurtz, 1992), were calling attention to children 'in need', children with 'educational and behavioural difficulties' and children with 'mental health problems'. They overlapped considerably.

Unfortunately, like that dividing Britain and America, a common language divided the agencies involved. Traditionally, health services were interested only if a child had a mental health problem, social services were interested only in children in need, and education services were interested only in children with emotional and behavioural difficulties. Children's developmental needs cannot be subdivided into different educational, social and health boxes without a similar dismembering of the child.

It was only in the early 1990s that the need to work across agencies achieved some political recognition as 'care in the community' was failing for lack of it. In 1993, as part of the Health of the Nation initiative, *Working Together for Better Health* (Department of Health, 1993) showed government recognition of health being dependent on 'healthy alliances' across agencies. To those using formulations which looked at the constitutional, family and environmental factors affecting children at their developmental stage this was nothing new, but it was quite a shift for medically based illness services.

Outcomes and economics

With a greater questioning of not just the organisation but also the legitimacy and funding of the welfare state, medical practice needed to be more systematic in its outlook in terms of interventions, outcomes, costs and effectiveness. The finite nature of resources became a given. In CAMHS there is a great deal of overlap in the work that team members do. This has raised challenging issues in terms of the economics of CAMHS organisation and costing. For example, with the development of community psychiatric nursing a briefer, task-focused way of working has provided the basis for a service that responds more readily and rapidly to children's difficulties.

Focus on health service management

The reorganisation of the National Health Service in the early 1990s had the expressed objective of making it more accountable to patient, taxpayer and government. An interest in the management of CAMHS became legitimate and sadly overdue as the problems were already well recognised (NHS Health Advisory Service, 1995a) (Box 2.1).

A strategic framework

This coalescence of historical factors led to a survey of service provision for the mental health of children and young people, which recognised the poor organisation of, and the poor coordination across, services (Kurtz et al, 1994). The publication the following year of *Together We Stand* (NHS Health Advisory Service, 1995a) provided a strategic framework for the organisation and comprehension of CAMHS. This has provided a springboard for CAMHS throughout the country to differentiate their four-tier functioning and clarify their operation at each of the tiers. However, by 1999 limited progress had been made (Audit Commission, 1999).

The inter-agency nature of CAMHS

The report from the Health Advisory Service both clarified the functioning of CAMHS and called attention to the fact that mental health problems in children and young people 'may arise from a young person's difficulties in coping with life, developmental difficulty, the impact of sensory handicap or an educational difficulty or from social difficulties'. These problems are caused by, and present, in all areas of a child's functioning. Parents, teachers, health visitors, social workers and so on have an important role in the maintenance of mental health. Education, social services, health services and the voluntary sector must work together, as children's mental health needs cannot be addressed separately. A multi-agency approach has to be at the core of services for children and young people with mental health needs. Health-based CAMHS have a major contribution to make to that multi-agency functioning.

Box 2.1 Problems in the management of CAMHS

- The purchaser–provider system put the buying power for services with general practitioners (GPs), who, on average, refer 4.5 children a year to CAMHS and therefore have a limited view of services. GPs therefore had to be wooed at the expense of social workers and education personnel with more experience and understanding of mental health problems in children.
- Needs assessments of young people's mental health needs had not been undertaken.
- The enthusiasms of therapists and teams traditionally drove interventions, which were often effective because of that enthusiasm. The concept of tailoring interventions to needs, rather than overriding therapeutic ethos, is a fairly new one in CAMHS.
- Multi-agency working within a service or team made the members of that team hostage to the fortunes of the managers of their agency. Social workers have been withdrawn from CAMHS all over the country, while other social services departments have demonstrated high levels of commitment to local CAMHS.
- Multi-disciplinary services and teams were easily rendered dysfunctional by pressures from disciplinary hierarchies. This contributed to the many institutional, professional and personal factors that disrupt the trust, mutual respect, sense of responsibility, role clarity, communication, commitment and clarity of purpose that a properly functioning multi-disciplinary service or team requires.
- Many services did not have operational policies or business plans, so their focus and functioning were unclear.
- Even within the health service, different professions still are frequently managed separately. For example, community nurses may have separate management from clinical psychologists, who may be separate from psychiatrists.
- In the competitive world of health provision, overlaps in desirable areas, and gaps in provision for the most difficult problems, were inevitable.
- Poorly managed services, which could not take a strategic view, were soon overwhelmed by the demanding nature of the work and became demoralised. The only defence then was long waiting lists and complex referral pathways that further demoralised them and alienated the community they purported to serve.
- User involvement and the resolution of the differing expectations of those involved with CAMHS remained a problem, although examples of innovative practice were available.

Developing a strategy

Certain CAMHS providers have been considerably assisted by forward-looking health authorities, which have invested in developing a comprehensive CAMHS strategy (Land, 1997) addressing key issues (Box 2.2). Such a strategy requires a champion or project leader to ensure it is transformed into a modern CAMHS rather than remaining a document gathering dust.

Box 2.2 The requirements of a strategy

- Multi-agency collaboration and service provision.
- Availability of information about services for young people and families.
- Support for those professionals who are the first point of contact for children and families.
- Promotion of mental health and prevention of mental health problems.
- Mental health service provision for the 16–25-year-old age range.
- Improved provision for children with learning disabilities who also have emotional, behavioural and mental health problems.
- Improved provision for children looked after by the local authority and leaving care.
- Involvement of young people and their families in the planning and provision of services.
- The provision of better-quality, and management control over, services through improved single-agency and joint commissioning.

Current context

The political context in which the health service will be operating in the future was outlined in the government white paper *The New NHS* (Department of Health, 1997a). This outlined changes which should be beneficial to recipients of CAMHS, such as:

- the integration of primary care and community services
- joint planning across agencies
- the possibility of pooled health and social service budgets
- an emphasis on co-terminus boundaries between health organisations and social services
- local authority membership of primary care organisations
- trusts having a statutory duty to collaborate.

The NHS Plan (Department of Health, 2000b) developed from this base. Although the National Service Framework for Mental Health applies primarily to adults of working age, some of the principles of health care delivery apply equally to children and young people (Department of Health, 2001d). A National Service Framework for Children is expected shortly and will provide guidelines for the development of CAMHS.

Commissioning by primary care organisations has the potential to ensure a more useful CAMHS design, as these organisations include senior representatives of the local authority. Primary care trusts that take responsibility for providing CAMHS as part of their mental health services or community children's services will have the difficult task of separating their commissioning from provider functions within one organisation. However, their agendas will be large and CAMHS will remain very small. A broader strategy may have to be visualised to encompass comprehensive CAMHS than will come into the purview of a primary care organisation. Joint-agency social care organisations are already appearing and are managing CAMHS in some parts of the country. The government's green paper *Our Healthier Nation* (Department of Health, 1998*b*) recognised the need for inter-agency working, so there is top-of-the-country ownership for such collaboration. Joint commissioning projects should now flourish, and blinkered agency managers flounder. CAMHS are increasingly subject to investigations and government directives, which should ensure that families will have the full range of skilled and competent professional support available to them.

The integration of the many current initiatives represents a considerable task (Box 2.3). Interventions are now expected to have an evidence base and directories of the evidence base are now appearing (Fonagy *et al*, 2002; Mental Health Foundation, 2002; Wolpert *et al*, 2002).

The tiered model

The tiered model is now generally accepted as the way to describe and understand CAMHS. A filter 'guards' entry to each tier. The first filter separates children, young people and their families from the first tier of professionals who work directly with them. Children with mental health problems and mental disorders primarily present their distress and behaviour to parents, teachers, health visitors and other workers within the community and a few to general practitioners. These professionals operate the second filter by deciding when it is necessary to involve a more specialist service, from Tier 2. It is here that a referral system may get in the way of good mental health. Those referred to a CAMHS often feel blamed, stigmatised, incompetent, bewildered and frightened; their mental health may be seriously assaulted by the referral process. The input of Tier 1 professionals may be considerably more helpful to the mental health of a young person and family than referral to Tier 2. Support of Tier 1 professionals therefore becomes a major task for CAMHS.

Tier 2 consists of specialist mental health workers – community psychiatric nurses, clinical psychologists, psychotherapists, child and adolescent psychiatrists, social workers and occupational therapists, who are usually organised in a CAMHS, working individually with young people and their families.

A service will also have a number of Tier 3 teams when a number of those professionals work together for a specific task, such as in a family therapy team or an eating disorders team.

Box 2.3 Current initiatives

- Combined National Planning and Priorities Guidance Objective 3 (NHS Executive, 1995) states: 'Improve provision of appropriate, high quality care and treatment for children and young people by building up locally based child and adolescent mental health services (CAMHS). This should be achieved through improved staffing levels and training provision at all tiers; improved liaison between primary care, specialist CAMHS, social services and other agencies; and should lead to users of the service being able to expect, (a) a comprehensive assessment and, where indicated, a plan for treatment without a prolonged wait, (b) a range of advice, consultation and care within primary care and Local Authority settings, (c) a range of treatments within specialist settings based on the best evidence of effectiveness, and (d) in-patient care in a specialist setting, appropriate to their age and clinical need.'
- The Audit Commission published its national survey findings in late 1999 (Audit Commission, 1999) and made recommendations for the future functioning of CAMHS, which included an increasing proportion of CAMHS time being devoted to the support of Tier 1 professionals.
- The social services 'Quality Protects' initiative.
- Local educational behaviour support plans.
- The establishment of youth offending teams.
- The establishment of Health Action Zones.
- The establishment of Education Action Zones.
- The establishment of drug action teams.
- The development of health improvement plans.
- The development of 'Sure Start' initiatives for the under-fives.
- The development of the Children's Fund for 5–13-year-olds.
- The development of 'Connexions' for 13–18-year-olds who appear to be becoming disaffected.
- The 'Valuing People' initiative for those with a learning disability (Department of Health, 2001c).
- The government's response to the Health Select Committee's *Report into Mental Health Services* (Department of Health, 2000a).
- *Promoting Children's Mental Health Within Early Years and School Settings* (Department for Education and Skills, 2001a).
- The *Special Educational Needs Code of Practice* (Department for Education and Skills, 2001b).

All of these initiatives are to be coordinated in *Building a Strategy for Children and Young People* (Children and Young People's Unit, 2001)

Tier 4 provides specialist services for a very small, but clearly defined, group such as those with sensory deficits or those requiring in-patient psychiatric care.

The advantages of this tiered approach to service provision are listed in Box 2.4.

Box 2.4 The advantages of a tiered approach

- The functioning of CAMHS is easier to understand; managing and evaluating services becomes clearer and simpler. The Audit Commission (1999) used the tiered system as a basis for its work on CAMHS.
- Resource input is related to complexity of need and appropriately filtered.
- The links required between tiers are clarified. Those between Tiers 2 and 3 and to Tier 4 services are often difficult because of geographical distances and the sometimes insular perspectives of Tier 4 facilities. Links between these, as espoused by the Care Programme Approach (Department of Health, 1990), are essential for integrated care pathways for young people requiring such specialist resources.
- Clarification of professional functioning gives confidence in role fulfilment in each tier. (Tier 3 teams often provide the glue that holds a service together.)
- Specific areas of service deficit are highlighted.
- Planning is facilitated because it is easier to identify areas where the service needs to develop or change its focus.
- Integration with other agencies that have such tiered structures is enabled. Indeed, staff such as educational psychologists and behaviour support staff do Tier 2 work in the education services, as do social workers in the social services. Similarly, each agency has its own Tier 3 and Tier 4 teams.

The future

Nationally, regionally and locally there are considerable pressures for change in CAMHS to ensure clearer functioning and inter-agency working. Resources are being made available nationally to drive these changes. Close cooperation between strategic health authorities, local authorities, health and social care trusts, primary care organisations, the courts, the Children and Families Court Advisory and Support Service (CAFCASS), the voluntary sector and other partner agencies will be required to ensure the child and adolescent population and their families benefit from those increased resources.

A common language across agencies is required that enables working together, to find a way of sharing information; this has been possible in child protection work (Department of Health *et al*, 1994; Department of Health & Welsh Office, 1995; Department of Health *et al*, 1999) and should not be an impossible task. There should be involvement of users and carers in the development of services in line with good clinical practice. Children and young people and their families should be able to follow pathways of care without encountering the barriers of inter-agency, inter-professional and inter-tier boundaries. The aim should be to provide a service that is accessible, multi-disciplinary, comprehensive, integrated with other agencies, accountable, and open to development and change (NHS Health Advisory Service, 1995*a*).

Great effort should also be made in finding ways of working with Tier 1 professionals that lighten their load and do not make them feel burdened with an extra task. There should also be moves towards the standardising of Tier 4 provision.

There are unprecedented resources coming into services for children and adolescents. For children and families to benefit there must be an overarching coordination of the many initiatives, which need to be owned by all agencies working with them. Extra resources in CAMHS will benefit children, young people and their families only if those services are properly commissioned, organised and managed.

CHAPTER 3

Structure, organisation and management of CAMHS

Ian Partridge, Nick Jones and Greg Richardson

'Here is Edward Bear, coming downstairs now, bump, bump, bump, on the back of his head, behind Christopher Robin. It is, as far as he knows, the only way of coming downstairs, but sometimes he feels that there really is another way, if only he could stop bumping for a moment and think of it. And then he feels that perhaps there isn't.'
A. A. Milne, *Winnie the Pooh*

Introduction

For a CAMHS to offer a service based on the principles described in *Together We Stand* (NHS Health Advisory Service, 1995*a*), geared to meeting the needs of the local community and its partner agencies, it must be clearly structured and efficiently managed (Box 3.1). A lack of attention to basic managerial principles often undermines the service provided, creating discord among, as well as pressure upon, individual professionals and teams. The resultant dysfunction can lead to

---

Box 3.1 Foundations for effective CAMHS

- A 'critical mass' of multi-disciplinary staff.
- Coordination and integration of professions and teams.
- Organisation within the tiered framework.
- The use of the individual and professional skills of all service members to their full potential.
- Clear lines of accountability, responsibility and supervision.
- A training and development programme for all disciplines.
- Prioritisation and management of work–load.
- Clear operational policies.
- Adequate administrative support.
- Overt inter-agency networks of communication.
- An agreed strategy.
- An interested and supportive management structure.
- A designated, consistent budget.
- Clinical governance.

---

inadequate service provision and low morale. Equally, a service that is perceived to be poorly organised and idiosyncratic is not going to attract investment. The starting point of the management structure must be the young person and family, not the requirements of the institution.

Management in tiers

The tiered model starts with the young person and family, whose first contact with mental health services will be at Tier 1. CAMHS must be structured around them to ensure their pathway of care through the service is as smooth as possible; CAMHS must therefore be structured in such a way that they start providing mental health input to young people through those with whom they have contact in their everyday lives. There is no reason why all CAMHS disciplines, with training and experience, cannot be involved in liaison and consultation with Tier 1 staff. Developing contacts, relationships and joint working with outside agencies will ensure that CAMHS are understood and used effectively by those providing a direct service to children and families.

At Tier 2, CAMHS must be organised for individual professionals to work with children and families, as this is a large percentage of the work undertaken by any CAMHS. They will require, in addition to the principles listed in Box 3.1, an awareness of the functioning and specialist skills of other disciplines inside and outside CAMHS, and the operational practices of partner agencies, so they can involve other disciplines and agencies as required by the children they see.

Tier 3 specialist teams provide an opportunity for certain CAMHS members to work together with a specific focus and to develop their skills in particularly complex areas. Tier 3 teams should offer training opportunities for all disciplines and model good interdisciplinary working. They require coordinators to perform the everyday administrative tasks of the team, to ensure work allocated to the team is appropriately managed and to provide a focal point for other members of the CAMHS.

Most CAMHS will not have a Tier 4 function and staff working at Tier 4 have specialist skills and often require their own discrete management structure.

A multi-disciplinary service

To work effectively at all tiers, a range of disciplines, skills and perspectives are required, so that children are offered a care package geared to their individual needs. A multi-disciplinary composition is therefore required that incorporates the skills necessary to address the clinical management of the wide and complex clinical problems presented (De Silva *et al*, 1995). Each discipline and all professionals have a responsibility to work in and provide support across all tiers. The effective working of each tier and the free movement of staff to work and provide support in each tier are vital to the functioning of a CAMHS as a whole. Within the service, each discipline will have its hierarchical and supervisory structure supporting the autonomous effectiveness of each profession.

Administrative staff are vital to the smooth and efficient running of any organisation. In addition to compiling and maintaining records for all aspects of the service, they may also take responsibility for the collection of statistical data that may be used for research and audit. These staff usually also work with patients and carers on the telephone and in the building, as well as the many professionals involved with patient care. Administrative staff are the direct link with the public and other agencies, and are often the first point of contact for both. To ensure the right skill mix, it is necessary to invest and train the staff not only in appropriate clerical and administrative skills but also in skills of diplomacy for this demanding and responsible area of work. The secretariat is often the service engine room, whose functioning is vital to the running of the ship. They should be recognised as such and at times of financial hardship, if regarded as an expendable ancillary service, such short-sightedness will bring the service to a juddering halt.

Management of the service

The professions and specialist teams within CAMHS generate many management roles. These roles must be recognised and differentiated, members of CAMHS taking on responsibility for different roles at different times, for example coordinator of a Tier 3 team as well as professional supervisor of a less experienced member of the same discipline and possibly professional lead. All meetings and teams within the service will require a chair or coordinator who ensures that the meeting or team deals with the business in hand (e.g. the management of referrals or professional supervision) and that action is taken on decisions (Hill, 1995). Staff meetings, which are geared to under-standing the work of the service, as opposed to decision-making meetings, may require a facilitator, who may be another staff member or someone from outside the service.

Within each profession there are hierarchies and the senior members have responsibility for the professional supervision and management of those more junior (e.g. senior doctors ensuring there is a duty rota of junior doctors).

The site on which the CAMHS is based will also require management, so that the accommodation and working environment of all staff members are attended to. The staff member who takes on this responsibility must be able to network well in the rest of the host organisation and have considerable skills in managing people.

The CAMHS management team

Overarching responsibility for the structure, organisation and operation of CAMHS is the task of a CAMHS management team. This team should consist of the senior members of all the professions working in the service and relevant members of the host organisation's management, so that they may address the tasks listed in Box 3.2.

The achievement of these tasks will require regular meetings, possibly monthly, to discuss clinical governance and financial matters, as well as performance. The annual budget for CAMHS should be clearly differentiated from other budgets in the trust. The budget will then require monitoring and managing (Gale, 1996). It may also be useful to have the budget further subdivided for different parts of CAMHS (e.g. the Tier 4 service and the Tiers 2 and 3 service). The budget will also be divided under separate headings, such as staff costs, travel, overheads and so on. A member of the host organisation's finance staff on the management group can be very helpful in understanding the financial situation. CAMHS that offer a specialist service, such as Tier 4 provision, may have the potential to generate income for the host organisation, which may be a useful lever to gain more resources for CAMHS and certainly to support the Tier 4 service. Close monitoring at year end (January–March) may reveal an under-spend which may enable the purchase of capital items before 31 March.

Box 3.2 Tasks of the CAMHS management team

- Monitoring the distribution of workload and service delivery.
- Ensuring clinical governance.
- Monitoring progress of the service against the strategy.
- Understanding, monitoring and containment of the service budget.
- Developing business plans to enhance the service.
- Ensuring partner agencies are involved in the operation of CAMHS.
- Ensuring the operational policy for the service is up to date.
- Ensuring all disciplines within CAMHS are represented.
- Bringing serious opportunities or threats to the notice of the host organisation.

Management within the wider host organisation

The CAMHS management team may be a clinical directorate in its own right, or a subgroup of a larger directorate. There has been considerable discussion as to whether CAMHS are best placed within the management of child health services or mental health services. CAMHS can be well managed and understood in both settings and such services often wish to stay where they are. Equally, CAMHS can be poorly understood and badly managed in both settings. The lesson seems to be to develop relationships with the existing management structure rather than leave it in hope of finding a more understanding master. CAMHS are managed within the burgeoning variety of trusts that are now developing: they may be part of a community and mental health trust, a mental health trust, a whole-district trust (if not with other mental health services), a primary care trust or a social care trust. They all have their advantages and disadvantages, although the last two have considerable inter-agency responsibility, which may be consonant with CAMHS.

Trusts are organised upon a continuum from general management to clinical directorates and the CAMHS management group must ensure it is fitted firmly into whichever organisational structure is in place. There is no reason why members of the CAMHS management group cannot take on wider management responsibilities (e.g. the nurse manager being on the trust board or the consultant psychiatrist being the clinical director of child health).

A CAMHS is only as strong as its weakest link. A service thatdoes not integrate its component parts into a cohesive whole will find itself in danger of fragmentation at times of pressure, retrenching to a position of low staff morale and complaints of lack of resources. A well-managed service has within it the recognition and support of all members of the team and will be fit for purpose in obtaining and using resources effectively.

CHAPTER 4

Clinical governance

Greg Richardson

'My own rules are very simple. Don't hurt nobody. Be nice to people.'
Sammy Davis Jnr

Definition

Clinical governance is a way of integrating financial control, service performance and clinical quality into the management of health services (Scally & Donaldson, 1998) and is the overarching principle of the management of CAMHS. It became an integral part of the health service with the publication of *A First Class Service* (Department of Health, 1998c), which described the methods by which the quality of services would be set, delivered and monitored. Concerns about medical practice have led to more specific publications on this topic (Department of Health, 2001f) and a commitment by the medical profession and the government to address this (NHS Executive, 2001).

Objectives

The objective of clinical governance is to provide clinical excellence to those served by the health services. In CAMHS this may be achieved by:

- moving the focus of CAMHS from finances and activity targets to quality
- safeguarding high standards of service delivery by creating an environment in which excellence in clinical care and awareness of current evidence will flourish
- continuously improving the quality of service delivered to children, young people and their families by developing the capacity to maintain high standards
- using failures and exemplars to increase the quality of care
- providing an organisational culture that encourages clear role definition within supportive teams and that discourages control by blaming.

Requirements

Good information technology

Information in the health services tends to focus on face-to-face contact with patients or on meeting waiting list targets. Such systems are clearly more geared to surgical services and do not meet the needs of a service working with families, carers and other agencies rather than individual patients. Performing a considerable amount of consultation, educational and supportive work at Tier 1 or involving Tier 3 teams dealing with different client groups does not fit current health information technology systems. The need for service-driven information systems geared to team working and Tier 1 support requires intensive work with information technology departments. Education is required for commissioners and host provider organisations, which, for all the development of hi-tech machinery for management, tend to operate from a late-19th-century view of a doctor-led, individual pathology treating service.

Access to evidence

All CAMHS members need to be involved in an active process of continuing professional development (CPD), which ensures they keep themselves up-to-date (Royal College of Psychiatrists, 2001). Yearly individual development reviews (IDRs) should be used to monitor this. Access to the internet should be available in all services as the modern alternative to libraries. Research and audit activities encourage service members' inquisitiveness about their practice.

Audit

An active multi-disciplinary audit programme should be in place (Hardman & Joughin, 1998). Initially these projects may be internally generated, but with input from involved agencies such as primary care organisations and user groups, outside interests can be incorporated into the annual audit cycle.

Staff training

Doctors generally have good access to training activities. Other disciplines tend to be poorly supported financially and the specificity of the clientele of CAMHS means that little training can take place in the locality. Methods of assessing training needs, and implementing them, should be part of the IDRs.

Time in which to review service

Mental health professionals need time out to review what they are doing to children, families and fellow professionals. Both community and in-patient teams require at least a half day every 6–12 months in which to take a more detached view of their work and to review service provision. Only when the nose is taken from the grindstone is it recognised that the nose is perhaps not the correct organ to be using and that the grindstone is not the most useful tool in these circumstances.

User involvement

User involvement is a notoriously difficult area in child and adolescent mental health as children, parents, teachers and social agencies often have conflicting views about what is an effective and helpful service and which of them is the user. Clinical practice means incorporating user and carer views into the management plan of every child. Formal reviews of the views of users of a particular part of the service (such as the participatory appraisal described in Chapter 8) can be part of an active audit programme.

Innovation

Innovation requires the development and encouragement of empowerment and facilitation skills. Having different professionals taking on coordinating and management roles in different parts of the service and in different Tier 3 teams encourages innovative and developmental thinking.

Team working and good working relations

Team working should be based on professional and individual role clarity, role confidence, role legitimacy, ownership of responsibility, commitment to children and families, collaborative agencies and colleagues, organisational clarity, high-level communication skills and, if possible, humour.

Effective professional regulation

Each profession has regulatory mechanisms (General Medical Council, 1998a). Service members should be close to each other's practice and use supervision, consultation and joint working to maintain professional standards.

Valuing and supporting staff

Staff will feel valued and supported if there is a strong team ethos. However, in the wider health service, there is often a perception that there is only ever interest when something goes wrong and that interest is investigative, not supportive, always looking for someone to blame. Schemes for the reporting of adverse incidents should investigate the way the organisational system is letting down health professionals, for all make mistakes and random blame encourages defensive and bureaucratic practice.

Effective coordination

All the very best efforts are wasted if they are not coordinated to a directed end. Every service and Tier 3 team requires a member to take responsibility for coordinating the efforts of that team so that it works efficiently. Their role should be defined in the operational policy.

Supportive and effective management

Good management encourages all of the above requirements for clinical governance while giving a sense of belonging and worth to the service. Hopefully the extremes of military dictatorship and abject disinterest and neglect are no longer features of the health service, but vigilance is necessary to protect services from their return.

Annual reports

All trust medical directors have to produce an annual clinical governance report. CAMHS within the trust are required to contribute to this as an integral part of performance management within the trust. The report may consider clinical governance matters in terms of meeting pre-determined standards (Royal College of Psychiatrists' Research Unit, 2001) or under topics such as those considered under separate headings below.

Standard setting and benchmarking, national and local

A CAMHS operational policy should integrate national and local requirements into its compliance with the local CAMHS strategy. Increasingly, standards are being set nationally (Royal College of Psychiatrists' Research Unit, 2001) and locally for CAMHS, which should play a part in generating their own, in order to engender investment and pride in the service.

Audit

Every CAMHS must have an active multi-disciplinary audit programme, which encompasses observational studies of how the service functions. This can lead on to the establishment of protocols and standards, which will then require regular monitoring. Evaluations of service and user perspectives also provide audit material, and so can affect service delivery.

Risk management

Many aspects of CAMHS delivery involve risk both to those using the service and to staff. Methods of recognising, estimating and managing those risks are part of everyday work and require increasing formalisation if services are not to be found deficient (Carson, 1990). Questions such as the safety of children in the waiting area, the protection of lone workers, the facility for speedy communication and the safety of self-harming adolescents are all topics that need to be addressed. If necessary, protocols should be developed. The risk management strategy should contain a process for learning from serious incidents to ensure that such incidents are monitored and investigated, that recommendations are implemented and that the changes required to prevent such an incident occurring again are monitored as part of the audit process.

Service development plans

Services should be developing all the time, informed by research evidence, national and local requirements, the results of audit processes, the risk management strategy and as a result of consumer surveys. New developments such as primary mental health workers or a new Tier 3 team, as well as new resources, require monitoring to ensure they are meeting their objectives in an efficient manner. Service development does not imply adding on new services to old, but giving up old methods of practice as new ones are shown to be more useful or expedient. Such change may not always be popular. The move to Tier 1 support, at the expense of referrals to Tier 2 or 3, is often not popular, especially with those who wish to dispose of a problem via a referral system and fax machine, or with service providers who consider their importance is measured by the length of their waiting list. Waiting lists are not an effective way of helping children and families. Overt prioritisation may be necessary to ensure those in most need or those most likely to respond to intervention are seen promptly when services are overwhelmed by referrals. For instance, general practitioners should be informed when a service is overtaxed and informed of priorities in terms of patient need. Then referrals can be closely monitored and those with insufficient information or those not meeting overt prioritisation criteria can be returned to referrers.

Training

The training and IDR needs of all staff require annual review to ensure appropriately trained, supported and competent staff are working in the service.

User involvement

Users' views may be sought as part of the audit process. Methods of regularly accessing user views require investigation and implementation.

CHAPTER 5

CAMHS and the law: the Children Act, the Mental Health Act, child protection, consent and confidentiality

Caroline Harris, Ian Partridge and Greg Richardson

'My nature is subdued
To what it works in, like the dyer's hand'
Shakespeare, Sonnet 140

Introduction

The law provides a framework for CAMHS, clarifies responsibilities and legitimises interventions. Legislation should provide a context in which the best interests of the young person and family can be attended to (Cullen, 1992).

Statutory and professional responsibilities demand a sound knowledge of the legal requirements when dealing with both children and individuals with mental illnesses. The two central pieces of legislation relevant to CAMHS are the Children Act 1989 and the Mental Health Act 1983; the latter is, however, under review and a new Mental Health Act is imminent. Their usage will be informed by the principle that the child's welfare is paramount, which underpins the Children Act 1989.

Children Act 1989

The Act represented a major rationalisation of the legal framework for dealing with children and identifies principles central to working with children and their families (Williams, 1992). All members of CAMHS should be aware of these principles (Table 5.1).

The Act goes on to identify principles that govern the courts and any court orders that relate to the care of children:

- the welfare of the child is paramount – Section 1(1)
- delay must be reduced and avoided – Section 1(1)

Table 5.1 Principles of the Children Act 1989

Principle	Description
Partnership	The importance of working together with children, families and other professionals. The notions of fairness, natural justice, openness, directness and honesty. Empathy and support should generate interventions.
Paramountcy	Any involvement with and interventions into the lives of children and their families must begin and end with the principle that the welfare of the child (physical, psychological, developmental and emotional) is paramount.
Assessment of risk	If there are concerns regarding the welfare of children, the local authority has a duty (Section 4) to investigate. This has implications for CAMHS professionals who have concerns about children's welfare.
Significant harm	In terms of welfare and risks, the central concept is that of significant harm and the risk of significant harm. This arises from both acts of commission and acts of omission (Adcock & White, 1998).
Planning	The Act states that there is always a need for multi-disciplinary and inter-agency cooperation and planning in working with children in need and at risk.
Communication	Identifiable networks of inter-agency communication, as well as communication with families, must be clarified.

- no order can be considered unless it is demonstrably better for the child than making no order at all
- account is taken of limiting legislation – Section 91(14).

The Act also introduces the Welfare Checklist (Box 5.1), which offers a framework for planning for children and their families. First, the child must be seen and understood in a developmental context. Second, the child must be seen in a relational and family context. Individual pathologising supports neither of these. Third, interventions must be both realistic and pragmatic, with reasonable aims and expectations, always striving for the least detrimental alternative and the intervention that will do not only the most good but also the least harm.

Mental Health Act 1983

The Mental Health Act 1983 applies to children and young people as well as adults. When they require interventions for the good of their mental health the choice between using the Mental Health Act or the Children Act may not be an easy one. However, the question of which Act to use arises only in the context of in-patient provision. The

Box 5.1 The Welfare Checklist

- The ascertainable wishes and feelings of the child, in light of age and understanding.
- The child's physical, emotional and educational needs.
- The likely effect on the child of any change in circumstances.
- The child's age, sex, background and any other characteristics the court considers relevant.
- Any harm the child has suffered or is likely to suffer.
- How capable each of the child's parents, or any other person in relation to whom the court considers the question to be relevant, is of meeting the child's needs.
- The range of powers available to the court under the Children Act in the proceedings in question.

guiding principles must be: clarity over the purpose of the intervention, and whether the child's interests are best safeguarded by recognising their primary status as a child or as mentally ill. After this has been assessed, consideration should be given to the least intrusive course of action. In terms of this professionals should:

- be aware of statutory provisions and have ready access to legal advice
- prioritise the welfare of the child and ensure treatment is clear, consistent and operating within a recognisable legal framework
- use the least restrictive option to ensure the child's safety and welfare.

Detention under the Mental Health Act 1983

The code of practice (Department of Health & Welsh Office, 1999) recognises the specific needs of children in terms of:

- being kept fully informed of their treatment
- taking into account their wishes (with due regard to age and understanding)
- taking into account the role of the parent or those with parental responsibility
- providing appropriate education.

In addition, the following will need to be considered:

- Who has parental responsibility and what are their views?
- If parents are separated, with whom does the child live, is there a residence order and should contact be made with both families?
- What is the child's capacity for decision making, offering consent to, or refusing, treatment?

- What should happen if the child or person with parental responsibility refuses to give consent to treatment?
- Could the child's needs be met via an alternative placement (i.e. provision by the social services department or the education service)?
- Emergency treatment can and should always be given if delay would be dangerous.

Most in-patient treatment, as well as community treatment, takes place on an informal basis, usually with the consent of both child and parents. However, consent is often primarily parental for, although a young person may be judged to be 'Gillick competent', Gillick competence is judged on the capacity to give consent, not withhold it (Richardson & Harris-Hendricks, 1996).

The sections of the Mental Health Act most often used within in-patient CAMHS are:

- Section 5.4 – whereby nursing staff are able to detain children wishing to self-discharge should they be concerned about their mental state, well-being and safety (this sections expires after four hours)
- Section 5.2 – another interim section instigated by medical staff, which stays in force for 72 hours and should precede conversion to a Section 2 or 3 order
- Section 2 – expiring after 28 days, this allows for assessment within an in-patient setting
- Section 3 – allows treatment to be renewed after three months (needs review)
- Section 117 – provides for a coordinating meeting before the discharge of any patient who has been detained under Section 3 of the Act and allows for multi-agency planning for care and treatment after discharge.

Child protection

CAMHS are not primarily child protection agencies. They are required to work at the interface of clinical practice and children's safety in both a proactive and a reactive manner. This requires the balancing of the responsibilities for the therapeutic management of children and their families with those of child protection. The complexities in maintaining this balance are best addressed by reference to the welfare of the child being at all times paramount. The assessing of the best interests of the child in such cases should always take place within a multi-disciplinary and multi-agency context (Department of Health *et al*, 1999).

Through their work, CAMHS have a role in informing and developing effective child protection strategies and interventions (Brophy, 2001).

Working with children and adolescents will invariably bring the CAMHS professional, of whatever discipline, into contact with issues of child protection. Both the 1989 Children Act and subsequent guidance (Home Office *et al*, 1991; Department of Health *et al*, 1994, 1999; Department of Health & Welsh Office, 1995) restated the need for disciplines and agencies to work together, in a network of communication and liaison, to ensure the welfare of the child remains paramount.

Suspicion, and disclosure, of abuse or neglect

The local area child protection committee (ACPC) will have clear guidelines for the management of child abuse and neglect, of which all CAMHS staff should be aware. Within CAMHS there should be clear lines of communication, responsibility and accountability for staff faced with child protection concerns. All staff should be aware of management of confidentiality, as differing criteria exist for different disciplines. The overriding duty (established by law) of the child's welfare being paramount means that, within CAMHS, the guiding principle is limited confidentiality. Significant harm or the risk of significant harm necessitates the activation of procedures designed to safeguard the welfare of the child, regardless of the fashion in which information was obtained.

Linked to this is the responsibility of managing the situation in such a fashion as to minimise any additional stress and distress caused to the child and family. The principles that apply are listed in Box 5.2.

In general, it is not the role of CAMHS professionals to undertake child protection investigations unless they are asked to perform a specific assessment following the instigation of child protection procedures.

Box 5.2 Principles of child protection

- Child protection is activated along established guidelines.
- Senior staff are consulted and informed.
- Information is presented to and discussed with the relevant agencies (e.g. social services, police).
- The child is kept fully and clearly informed of what is happening.
- The family are informed as soon as is safe for the child.
- The child is never put in more danger by the intervention.
- Clear, detailed and, where possible, contemporaneous notes are kept.
- Attendance at any subsequent inter-agency meeting is prioritised.

Inter-agency cooperation

The importance of inter-agency cooperation can be seen in the number of guidelines and publications with 'working together' in the title. It is important that practical steps are taken by CAMHS to operationalise this process beyond attendance at occasional case conferences. The tiered system gives a clear framework for so doing and offers a mechanism whereby CAMHS can contribute fully and effectively to child protection.

Tier 1

Working with and offering support to Tier 1 workers are a vital part of CAMHS function, and child protection is no exception. Some Tier 1 workers (e.g. social workers) have primary responsibility for child protection in terms of its investigation and safeguarding the interests of the child. Advice, consultation and support from a CAMHS professional regarding psychological impact and sequelae, and the placing of child abuse within a systemic and developmental context, can enable this process to be more effective. A wider supervisory and advisory function may exist in work with other Tier 1 professionals.

Work in child abuse and protection is emotionally draining and can have an impact upon individual professionals and professional networks, as well as the children and their families. The CAMHS professional may be able to offer support and understanding to such professionals, as well as a sense of detachment from the decision-making process.

Tier 2

CAMHS workers operating individually at Tier 2 may be involved in working with children and families where child protection issues are of either direct importance or indirect concern. In such work, multi-agency liaison and effective communication networks must exist, so that each agency understands its role and the questions it has to address. Knowing who's who in social services and the police, as well as developing relationships with these agencies, enables the effective management of child protection processes. Being aware of guidelines, responsibilities and what is expected of various agencies and professionals ensures that work can be performed without recourse to panic; it also offers a calmer background for both child and family.

Tier 2 professionals may also be involved in post-investigation therapeutic work with children and families. The issue of therapeutic work during investigation and possible prosecution can be problematic; however, the clinical needs of children in terms of their emotional, psychological and physical well-being must be carefully weighed in terms of the responsibility to prioritise the welfare of the child.

Tier 3

CAMHS may develop particular Tier 3 services, to work in the area of child protection on a reactive and preventive level. Examples include risk assessment teams, therapeutic group work, family therapy and parent–child relationship groups. In all these areas, liaison with other agencies must be established to avoid isolated working and clearly to establish their task in the management of the situation. Such specialist teams may also have an input to inter-agency training initiatives, as well as having representation upon the ACPC.

Tier 4

Specialist services such as in-patient units may provide a setting wherein disclosure of, or awareness of, child abuse occurs – the principles outlined above also apply here. It may also be that children who develop serious mental health problems have experienced some form of neglect or abuse that is pertinent to their present condition and may affect planning for them. Equally, the skilled assessment of abuse in the context of mental illness may be a function of CAMHS. In this area, the centrality of multi-disciplinary and multi-agency planning and working cannot be overstressed.

Consent

Consent must be informed to be valid, hence the use of the single word 'consent'. Consent is a complex issue when working with children and young people, as it applies to parents as well as their children. Fortunately, guidance is provided by the Department of Health (2001e). The recent introduction of the Human Rights Act (see below) also has some important implications in this area for health care professionals.

Definition

Consent is defined in the Mental Health Act 1983 Code of Practice (Department of Health & Welsh Ofice, 1999) as:

'The voluntary and continuing permission of the patient to receive a particular treatment, based on an adequate knowledge of the purpose, nature, likely effects and risks of that treatment including the likelihood of its success and any alternatives to it. Permission given under any unfair or undue pressure is not consent.' (Para. 15.13)

For consent to be valid, four components are required:

* adequate information needs to be provided to the individual
* the individual must have capacity to give consent
* there must be an absence of coercion

- available alternatives to the intervention offered need to be outlined.

Consent can be withdrawn at any point during the intervention and 'the [competent] patient's right of choice exists whether the reasons for making that choice are rational, irrational, unknown or even non-existent' (*Re T* [1992] 4 All ER 649, cited in Lilley *et al*, 2001). The exception to this right of accepting or refusing treatment is laid out within the provisions of Part IV of the Mental Health Act 1983.

Competence

A recent document (Department of Health, 2001*a*) on seeking consent when working with children clearly outlines the area of competence. Adults (18 years or over) and young people (16–18 years) are presumed to be competent unless one of the three following difficulties are evident (Department of Health, 2001*b,e*):

- The individual is unable to take in and retain the information necessary to make the decision, especially with respect to the likely consequences of having or not having the treatment.
- The individual is unable to believe the information.
- The individual is unable to weigh the information, balancing risks and needs.

For children (under 16 years of age) there is no presumption of competence and competence therefore must be assessed. Consent can be given by the child or young person, the parent, the local authority (if the child is in care) or by a court. The Department of Health offers advice to children and young people on consent (Department of Health, 2001*a*). If the child consents to treatment and is assessed by a health care professional to be competent, then there is no need, legally, to obtain the parent's consent. However, it is seen as good practice and preferable to gain both child and parental consent when at all possible and to involve all those close to the child in the decision-making process (Department of Health, 2001*b*). The Gillick ruling (Appeal Cases, 1986) states that a competent young person should have 'sufficient understanding and intelligence to enable him or her to fully understand what is being proposed', understanding the risks and benefits of the intervention beyond immediate discomforts.

However, there are additional complexities in assessing competence. The Mental Health Act Code of Practice (Department of Health & Welsh Office, 1999) also states (in para. 15.10) that decisions must be made in relation to the particular treatment, that capacity can vary over time and that all assessments of capacity should be fully recorded. Moreover, the degree of capacity required varies according to the

---

> **Box 5.3** Areas for assessment of competence in children and young people
>
> - Ability to understand choice and consequences of choice.
> - Willingness and ability to make choice.
> - Understanding of purpose, nature and effects of intervention.
> - Understanding of no intervention or alternative interventions, including attendant risks.
> - Freedom from pressure.
> - Reason for absence of parental consent.

seriousness of the treatment for which consent is being sought, and so increased capacity needs to be demonstrated with increased seriousness of the decision.

Assessing competence

There are no formalised assessment procedures for the evaluation of competence. However, criteria from the practice guidelines for clinical psychologists (British Psychological Society, 2001) are consistent with guidelines from the British Medical Association (2001) and and provide a useful outline for assessing the competence of children and young persons relevant to all health care professionals (see Boxes 5.3 & 5.4).

Human Rights Act 1998

The Human Rights Act, adopted by the UK Parliament in October 2000, seeks to ensure that laws, practices and procedures comply with the rights set out in the European Convention on Human Rights (ECHR). The ECHR aims to protect human rights and fundamental freedoms, and to maintain and promote the ideals and values of a democratic society. The European Human Rights Act consists of 18 articles and six protocols, but not all of these are incorporated into UK law. One notable article missing is Article 13, which guarantees 'an effective remedy before national authority', and therefore compensation for the violation of an individual's human rights will have to be decided in Strasbourg (MIND, 2001).

The introduction of the Human Rights Act has and will continue to have a major impact on the development of mental health law and practice, as it requires all public authorities (which include health and social care agencies) to act in a manner that is compatible with the ECHR. Individuals who have had or may have had their rights violated within the mental health services can therefore take legal action against the relevant authority. Many of the rights found in the ECHR have a direct impact on the provision of care for people with mental health

Box 5.4 Good practice in relation to consent and the assessment of competence (sources include British Psychological Society, 2001; Department of Health, 2001*a*)

Principles
- Although parental consent is not legally required if a child is assessed by a health care professional to be competent and the child consents to treatment, it is preferable to gain both child and parental consent.
- If the views of the parent differ from the child and this cannot be resolved through negotiation, the primary obligation is always the child's interests.
- Informed consent is a process, needing continual review.
- If a child is not considered competent, clinical work should support active participation in decision making by giving clear information and eliciting the child's views. This is heavily emphasised in the recent Department of Health document (2001*a*).

Standards of good practice
- Information should be provided at the appropriate developmental level of the child. The amount of information given should be appropriate to the length and nature of the intervention.
- Children should always be informed of the purpose of the work and the practical arrangements involved, even if their consent has not been obtained.
- Negotiating different views is common when obtaining informed consent. Consent may need to be gained in a series of steps, in which case each stage should be recorded in the notes.
- When a child consents to treatment but the parent does not consent, then: record clearly the assessment of the child's competence, reasons why the parent has not provided consent and the agreement reached with the child concerning confidentiality; provide the child with written confirmation of the arrangements made; discuss the case in supervision or with senior colleagues and record this in the notes.
- The rare situation of a child assessed to be competent refusing an intervention will best be resolved in a multi-disciplinary setting. Supervision and consultation with other colleagues are essential. Overriding a child's wishes is justifiable only in circumstances where there is a significant threat to life or a threat of long-term significant harm and where the benefits of the intervention are relatively clear, for example when the withholding of antipsychotic medication in an early-onset psychosis could contribute to avoidable developmental damage. Legal advice or court approval may be necessary in these situations, especially when the parent refuses consent as well. For instance, if a non-compliant young person with anorexia refuses food, feeding will need to take place under Section 3 of the Mental Heath Act in order to protect both the child and the staff.
- The more complex and problematic decisions should always be made with multi-disciplinary input.
- Consent is required for sharing or obtaining information from other professionals or agencies. Again, if the child's best interests override consent, then this should be documented.
- Regular supervision and peer review are recommended.

problems. Those agencies and professionals involved in such care need to review their practices and procedures to ensure they lie within the ECHR (Sainsbury Centre for Mental Health, 2000). This has the potential for increasing good practice and ensuring respect for individual rights.

Consent

Articles 3 and 8 of the ECHR, 'freedom from torture and inhuman or degrading treatment or punishment' and 'the right to respect for private and family life, home and correspondence', respectively, have implications for ensuring consent of individuals is obtained before that individual undertakes medical treatment or psychological assessment, investigation or intervention (Henson, 2000; Lilley et al, 2001). In a law case in Denmark (X v. Denmark, 1983, 32 DR 282 – cited in Outhwaite, 2000) the court found experimental or non-consensual medical treatment was shown to be in breach of Article 3. This can be seen to be a precedent for including all health care interventions, including psychological ones. Absence of obtaining consent or acting in the best interests of an individual will be breaching Article 8 if the exceptions laid out in the article are not met (Outhwaite, 2000). If informed consent is not obtained, or incapacity is not demonstrated and acting in the best interests of an individual is not indicated, then the health care professional in question would be in breach of Article 3 or 8 of the ECHR and could be charged as such in a UK court of law. Furthermore, it is vital for all health care professionals to be able to show that they have made methodical and continuous documentary records. It is important to note that this relates to both clinical and research work.

Confidentiality

Article 8 of the ECHR, 'the right to respect for private and family life, home and correspondence', has clear implications on confidentiality of information acquired through professional practice or research (Gostin, 2000; Lilley et al, 2001). This implies a responsibility for the protection of the privacy of individuals or organisations about whom information is collected or held. Part of the wide interpretation of Article 8 includes cases (MS v. Sweden, 1997, 3 BHRC 248; Z v. Finland, 1998, 25 EHRR 371 – cited in Outhwaite, 2000) where the court found an individual's right to privacy (under Article 8) was breached through the lack of protection of medical notes and other data. This has clear implications and relevance for health care records. A health care professional who does not maintain confidentiality without the individual's consent, or who breaks confidentiality without just cause, will be in breach of Article 8 of the ECHR, and could face charges brought in a UK court.

CHAPTER 6

Multi-disciplinary working

Ian Partridge, Greg Richardson, Geraldine Casswell
and Nick Jones

'All pigs are equal ...'
George Orwell, *Animal Farm*

Introduction

Effective CAMHS are based on multi-disciplinary working. However, while such working is a fundamental strength of practice, it can cause division and discord if there is not a clear understanding of its nature and tensions. The egalitarian models of multi-disciplinary teams in the 1970s have moved on. The roles of CAMHS members are defined not only by their professional training but also by their individual interest, development and expertise. A well-functioning team can be stronger than the sum of its parts, but requires commitment from individuals to a team ethos and a preparedness to recognise the professional skill, experience and interest of other disciplines. As with families, boundaries and roles need clarity, communication needs to be open and an ability of members to contain anxiety is essential. CAMHS differ from each other both in numbers and in disciplinary composition, so a systemically informed approach to team dynamics and personal and professional relationships is required for successful team working. In moving away from a doctor-led, illness-based model, the central issue is that of the integration of all disciplines in a fashion that values, legitimises and supports both the parts and the whole (Box 6.1).

One reason that Tier 3 working is important within CAMHS is that it requires joint working across disciplines and thereby entails a development of multi-disciplinary familiarity and understanding.

The team will function badly if there are unbreachable gulfs between members (Box 6.2), but equally if there is uncritical consensus. It Many teams of professionals who employ a systemic and developmental approach to their clinical work seem to behave as if such mechanisms for understanding do not apply to them (Kraemer, 1994). These issues do not just go away if they are not discussed; in the service, just as in the 'conflict avoiding' family, tensions find a way of surfacing, usually to the detriment of the children for whom services are being provided.

Box 6.1 Principles of multi-disciplinary working

- Specific disciplinary functions are clearly delineated and understood within the CAMHS.
- Each discipline is involved at all tiers.
- Inter-disciplinary training.
- Agreed operational policies for teams and services that are evolved and developed in a multi-disciplinary forum.
- Forums for multi-disciplinary discussion of clinical and organisational issues.
- Professional supervision within individual disciplines and access to multi-disciplinary supervision in a clear management structure.
- Administrative support.

The concept of 'disciplinary autonomy' is vital for CAMHS, as each discipline has its own hierarchy and is accountable for its own work with children, young people and their families. Traditionally, there has been a view that the buck of each discipline's work stops on the consultant psychiatrist's desk. It is important that this myth is erased from the thinking of all agencies and all employers, as well as individual disciplines and professionals within CAMHS. Teams will be undermined if individual members are too insecure or precious about their status and ultimate power and responsibility is given to one profession. To function effectively, each professional within a CAMHS must have role adequacy, role legitimacy and role support (NHS Health Advisory Service, 1995*a*).

Box 6.2 Tensions in multi-disciplinary working

- Clinical overlap in the skills of the differing professionals.
- Differences in skill levels and diversity between disciplines.
- Differentials in salary.
- Differentials in both professional and social status.
- The influence of agencies outside CAMHS that may have little under-standing of, or respect for, the multi-disciplinary model.
- Inter-disciplinary rivalries and resentments rooted in historical, personal and professional experiences.
- Differing training perspectives in different disciplines (multi-disciplinary training is in its infancy).
- Different disciplines having different roles, responsibilities and priorities, leading to varying notions of professional 'good practice' (e.g. confidentiality).
- Hierarchies of regard depending on personal attributes as much as professional ones.

Role adequacy

The World Health Organization's (1992) categories of emotional and behavioural disorders in version 10 of the *International Classification of Diseases* (ICD–10) would appear to make the role of CAMHS quite simple by clearly defining psychiatric disorders, which CAMHS should be able to assess and manage. However, it is not only medically trained professionals who can assess and treat these conditions and hence they are wisely called 'mental disorders'. In children the term 'mental health problem' (see Glossary), which has an even wider definition, has come to prominence. Epidemiological work suggests that between 5% and 15% of primary-school-aged children have emotional or behavioural psychiatric disorders that interfere with social or educational functioning (Cox, 1994). Where the criterion of need for treatment has been used, the estimates are nearer the lower end of this range (Vikan, 1985), but such numbers are still beyond the individual interventions of CAMHS. All CAMHS members therefore require skills in the management of young people, consultation and preventive work as well as in the many modes of therapeutic intervention. Maintenance and development of the core skills requires ongoing training and supervision if role adequacy is to be maintained.

Role legitimacy

This is the area where the vexed questions of traditional roles within a health service, medical responsibility, leadership and anxiety management arise. Psychiatrists may be considered fortunate in that they are well-paid, highly trained members of a profession which, despite recent publicity, remains highly valued by the public. They are in short supply and are members of one of the most powerful trades unions in the country, the British Medical Association. This allows them to command public respect and a revered position in the health service. Like parents in a similar position, they have considerable rights, but with those go some heavy responsibilities. Other disciplines may not be so fortunate and may find the struggle for legitimacy to be a slightly more uphill one – they may appear, like the identity-seeking adolescent, to be in search of respect and a desire to be taken seriously. This demonstrates a serious lack of understanding of their maturity in their roles, which will be recognised only if those roles are clearly defined, respected and rewarded.

Traditional roles

Traditionally, consultant psychiatrists are viewed as the ultimate medical authority and hence the people to whom others turn when uncertain, and in view of their length of training, this may be legitimate. In CAMHS, problems are rarely purely medical, so the 'ultimate authority' of the consultant is far more questionable. This is recognised in that some clinical psychologists and nurses are consultants. The traditional role also means that the psychiatrist will be expected to take on management roles in terms of strategic development and operational monitoring of CAMHS. Such a role, which may be formalised in the post of clinical director, provides a complex task in view of the different professions and personalities involved, and the need to maintain networks in the organisation's management structure. There is no reason why other professions cannot take on such directorial roles, but it will be very difficult for them to operate without the cooperation of the psychiatrists.

Medical responsibility

The concept of medical responsibility engenders more anxiety in psychiatrists and ill feeling in other disciplines than any other. Psychiatrists are not responsible for patients seen by other members of teams or services of which they are members. They are not responsible for young people who are discussed with them, although their advice must not be negligent. They do not have to vet every referral into their service, as this delays assessment and treatment, and is negligent in its own right. Most young people referred to CAMHS demonstrate their distress in their behaviour and one cannot be medically responsible for behaviour unless it is clearly caused by a medical condition. Referrals come to a team, so the most appropriate member of CAMHS can deal with that referral. CAMHS members are trained professionals who can work with young people and their families without constant oversight from a psychiatrist. There will be considerable overlap in the work of professionals within a CAMHS and for a multi-disciplinary team to operate effectively disciplinary functions should be recognised without the creation of a false hierarchy of regard for any one discipline.

Medical responsibility is 'professional competence, good relationships with patients and colleagues and observance of professional ethical obligations' (General Medical Council, 1995). Indeed, the term 'medical responsibility' no longer appears to be used in General Medical Council literature.

Leadership

The traditional expectations of psychiatrists may lead to an automatic assumption of their leadership. Such expectations may be unrealistic in that a particular psychiatrist may not have leadership qualities or may misunderstand the leadership role, leading to the rest of the CAMHS resenting the psychiatrist's assumption of this role. The effective multi-disciplinary functioning of the CAMHS will then be disrupted. Leadership must be distinguished from management, coordination, supervision and professional hierarchy, all of which are easier to define and the place of each professional within them clearer. Leaders are primarily required at times of change or uncertainty. They may therefore be defined as the person to whom other members of CAMHS go when they are worried about something – the 'anxiety sump' or, as Napoleon put it, 'a dealer in hope'.

Five styles of leadership are described (Gatrell, 1996): those who tell, those who sell, those who consult, those who participate and those who delegate. In professional hierarchies, telling may be appropriate, but for effective team functioning participation and delegation are required.

Anxiety management

The maxim for all those working in CAMHS should be the first lines of Britain's favourite poem:

'If you can keep your head while all about you
Are losing theirs and blaming it on you'.

'Not keeping your head' perfectly describes the responses of adults to young people's very difficult behaviour when they are bereft of any idea of what to do to manage the situation. The idea of 'illness' provides a convenient repository for a lack of understanding. Finding calm, structural solutions among a seething, projecting, emotional maelstrom is the task of any CAMHS professional as the ultimate consultative task. The service member who can do this best and to whom other members of the team turn in such situations is the key member of the service and may even be the leader.

Role support

The support to provide a service comes from the organisation in which the professionals work. Such support arises from the disciplinary structure, the multi-disciplinary team and the host organisation's management structure. Role support is very variable in different settings and the professional who is unable to obtain it must consider whether it is tenable to continue to work in such an organisation. Professionals often feel overloaded by conflicting clinical and managerial pressures. Methods of addressing this are described for adult psychiatrists (Kennedy & Griffiths, 2000), who are steadily catching up with the innovative practices of child and adolescent mental health professionals.

The roles of individual disciplines

Clinical child psychologists

Following an undergraduate psychology degree, postgraduate quali-fication is obtained in clinical psychology. It is usual for a year of relevant practical experience to be sandwiched between the two. Specialisation follows generic training and the clinical psychologist will have:

'a holistic view of a child and the child's behaviour and relationships in the contexts in which they occur. Knowledge of normal and abnormal child development, and of the wide range of psychological factors, which influence children and their families, is utilised in the assessment of childhood problems.' (British Psychological Society, 1993)

Trained in the administration of psychometric testing, clinical psy-chologists are able to offer a range of assessment and therapeutic options and have a role in working in all tiers of a CAMHS.

Community psychiatric nurses (CPNs)

The majority of CPNs will be registered mental nurses (RMNs), although this training offers little specific in terms of the theory and practice of working with children and their families. As a result of this there is a need for post-qualification training in relevant areas. Specialist courses have evolved, such as the ENB 603 course in child and adolescent mental health. CPNs operate as key members of a CAMHS and are able to offer a prompt response as well as key assessment and treatment options. It is important that CPNs work in all tiers of the CAMHS and are not used solely as Tier 2 professionals.

In-patient psychiatric nurses

Nurses working in the Tier 4 in-patient service will include RMNs, some of whom will have obtained post-qualification ENB 603 training, nurses who are generally trained and qualified, and untrained nursing assistants. The in-patient nursing staff are the key and backbone to any in-patient unit offering skilled nursing care and a range of therapeutic inputs to the young people and their families under their care. It is possible that in-patient staff may have a role in Tier 3 teams that are closely associated with their Tier 4 function.

Child, adolescent and family psychiatrists

Medically qualified, they will specialise in general psychiatry before completing Membership of the Royal College of Psychiatrists; a further three years of specialist training specifically in child and adolescent psychiatry will follow before they achieve consultant status. The role of the psychiatrist in CAMHS has been described (Black, 1996).

The child psychiatrist may deliver social, psychological and medical treatments. Under the Mental Health Act 1983, consultant psychiatrists, having obtained Section 12 approval, may be required to detain and treat psychiatrically ill young people. For in-patients the medical responsibility will lie with the consultant. Psychiatrists should work within all tiers of a CAMHS.

The position of the psychiatrist in the team is often a source of difficulty and conflict. There has been considerable debate about what psychiatrists should spend their time doing (Goodman, 1998), as they are an expensive resource who should be directed to maximum effect. Psychiatrists spend longer in training than most other mental health professionals, and this allows them to become skilled at the assessment and management of mental disorders. The fact that such skills may overlap in part with other professionals' skills does not impair either the psychiatrist's or other disciplines' role adequacy. In the National Health Service generally, more money is allocated to the postgraduate and in-service training of doctors than that of any other profession, so the potential to maintain that role adequacy may be greater than for any other mental health profession.

Social workers

Social workers are usually employed by the local social services department and attached to the CAMHS. This means they will be independent of the trust administering the CAMHS and have distinct line management and accountability. Such an attachment should, where possible, be full time and exclusive, so that specialist skills can be developed and the CAMHS can operate in a fully integrated multi-disciplinary fashion. Social workers are often but not always graduates, who undertake postgraduate training that results in the Diploma in Social Work or the Certificate of Qualification in Social Work (CQSW); they often go on to obtain masters degrees. Their training is generic; however, there is the scope for some specialisation during training. Social workers may follow up their training with post-qualification training in specialist areas.

Social workers have statutory responsibilities in the field of child protection. Their work is structured by the rule of law, specifically the Children Act 1989 and the Mental Health Act 1983 (some will be 'approved social workers' under the terms of the latter) in terms of their responsibilities with regard to the rights of children and their families. Social workers should work within all tiers of the CAMHS.

Other disciplines

The professions highlighted above represent the core of any CAMHS: with the lack of any of those disciplines, it is difficult for a CAMHS to function coherently. However, there are a range of other disciplines that can be successfully integrated into a CAMHS and have valuable insights to offer to the mental health needs of children and families. Examples include occupational therapists, child psychotherapists, family therapists, and music, art and drama therapists as well as educationalists (teachers and educational psychologists).

CHAPTER 7

Evidence-based practice

Juliette Kennedy and Ian Partridge

'The greatest obstacle to discovering the truth is being convinced that you already know it.'
Anon

Introduction

The underlying philosophy of evidence-based practice is that therapeutic interventions should be rational, measurable and observed to benefit their recipient (Laugharne, 1999). This leads to an attempt to standardise the way all health care workers make clinical decisions, with a strong emphasis on using the best evidence available from research:

'The aim is to see that Research and Development (R&D) becomes an integral part of health care, so that managers and practitioners find it natural to rely on the results of research in their day to day decision making. ... Strongly held views, based on belief rather than sound information, still exert too much influence in health care. In some instances knowledge is available but is not being used, in other situations additional knowledge needs to be generated from reliable sources.' (Peckham, 1991)

In this statement the government set an agenda that obliges all health care professionals to use evidence-based approaches to their clinical decision-making.

Access to evidence

The majority of research evidence is unevaluated (see Figure 7.1). It is also of enormously variable quality. In order to find an answer to many clinical dilemmas, this unevaluated evidence will still need to be read and interpreted by the practising clinician. The National Institute for Clinical Excellence (NICE) has issued some evidence-based guidelines as directives for clinical practice, in order to try to prevent the usual time lag between some clinicians determining and developing best practice, and everyone else catching up. However, only a small part of the service will be standardised by central direction. Evidence-based practice is 'the conscientious, explicit and judicious use of, current best evidence, in making decisions about the care of individual patients'

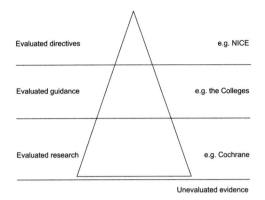

Figure 7.1 Access to research evidence.

(Sackett *et al*, 1997) and it is generally assumed that best evidence comes primarily from scientific research. This maintains the fundamental principle that evidence from clinical research studies is more trust worthy than reasoning from basic physiology, pathology, psychology or clinical intuition (Evidence-Based Medicine Working Group, 1992). Research, however, has its own objectives (see Box 7.1); it may point the direction of practice but it rarely answers a question completely for one particular patient.

Clinical practice

Views about evidence-based practice have tended to become polarised. Critics typically caricature its enthusiasts as research evangelists who fail to appreciate the complexity of everyday practice, and overlook the wisdom of experienced clinicians. Advocates of evidence-based practice view its opponents as 'Luddites' who have overvalued ideas about their clinical acumen (Geddes & Harrison, 1997). However, a balance has to be struck in clinical decision-making between the following factors (Graham, 2000):

- the best available *external clinical evidence* from systematic research that is relevant to the child and family's problem

---

Box 7.1 The functions of research (adapted from Bury & Mead, 1998)

- Generating new knowledge.
- Providing 'generalisable' results (i.e. that can be applied to a wider population of similar patients).
- Challenging current practice.
- Informing policy and service delivery.

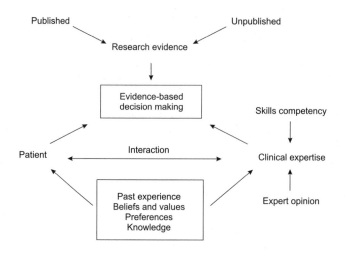

Figure 7.2 Sources of information needed for clinical decision-making (from Bury & Mead, 1998, reprinted by permission of Elsevier Ltd).

- *individual clinical expertise* (i.e. the skills and judgement clinicians acquire from the experience of seeing patients) and in particular the skills in diagnosis and in understanding the context in which the family's problem has occurred
- an appreciation of the *child and family's preferences and rights* when making decisions about their care.

Good clinicians will use each of these components in an integrated way. One alone is not enough (Figure 7.2). Without clinical expertise, practice risks becoming tyrannised by external evidence, as even excellent external evidence may be inappropriate for the individual patient (Sackett *et al*, 1997). Patient preference may override research evidence in some cases, for example if the family declines to engage in family therapy, despite this intervention being supported by the best research evidence for their problem. The service would then need to consider alternative options, taking into account any other available external evidence.

'The sharp distinction between external evidence and clinical expertise can have the serious disadvantage of conveying a message that clinical experience does not produce evidence. In common terms the average child and adolescent mental health worker is likely to define "evidence" broadly, as any information useful in making a clinical decision. Most clinicians would think of several relevant clinical experiences with similar patients as reasonably strong evidence.' (Graham, 2000)

There is a need to integrate all available information in clinical decision-making (Box 7.2); data obtained from a clinical assessment

---

Box 7.2 Evidence-based decision-making (Rosenberg & Donald, 1995)

- Formulate a clear clinical question from the patient's problem.
- Search the literature for relevant articles (using Medline and other databases).
- Critically appraise the evidence for its validity and usefulness.
- Implement useful findings in clinical practice.
- Evaluate, via clinical audit, the impact of the change in practice (Bury & Mead, 1998).

---

should be combined with information derived from generalisable research, to form a theory about a particular young person in a particular family. The theory can then be tested, by checking with other sources of information or by trying an intervention and seeing if the outcome is consistent with the theory. If the theory is correct, an appropriate intervention will ameliorate the problem (Graham, 2000). Clinical expertise is the essential tool for the efficient gathering of case evidence; it is necessary in integrating case evidence with external evidence from research, applying that which is relevant to the problem in hand, engaging the family and integrating their views and preferences. Only then can an effective management plan be formulated.

Clinical questions are produced from the clinical dilemmas that arise when constructing management plans for patients or when attempting to improve an element of the service. A common question might be along the following lines:

'For this young person with anxiety what are the possible effects of cognitive–behavioural therapy versus relaxation training and therefore which therapy should be offered?'

Increasingly, the public are informing themselves, particularly through the internet, of the evidence available from research. They may be basing their choices about their own and their family's health care on this information (Wright *et al*, 1999). Professionals need to be aware of the latest research, but importantly they need to develop a facility for both critical selection and appraisal. Critical appraisal is a complex skill that requires practice. Not all clinicians are interested in doing this intensive study in the face of the time constraints of clinical practice.

Evidence-based resources

There is increasing interest in 'evidence-based resources' (Guyatt *et al*, 2000), where experts in critical appraisal produce summaries of important new studies they have analysed which can be quickly read by others. The *Journal of Evidence-Based Mental Health* and the FOCUS

Box 7.3 Article selection guide (from Oxman *et al*, 1993)

Therapy
- Was the assignment of patients to treatment randomised?
- Were all the patients who entered the trial accounted for at the end?

Diagnosis
- Was there an independent, blind comparison with a control group?
- Did the patient sample include an appropriate spectrum of the sort of patients to whom the diagnostic test will be applied in clinical practice?

Harm
- Were there clearly identified comparison groups that were similar with respect to important determinants of outcome (other than the one of interest)?
- Were the outcomes and exposures measured in the same way in the groups being compared?

Prognosis
- Was there a representative patient sample at a well-defined point in the course of the disorder?
- Was follow-up sufficiently long and complete?

---

initiative of the Royal College of Psychiatrists are beginning to produce evidence-based briefings.

Other options include adapting national guidelines for local implementation where these are available, or a member of the service looking at the primary studies and any systematic reviews (Box 7.3) and producing guidelines or protocols for all team members to use at a local level.

Clinical effectiveness and cost-effectiveness

Clinical effectiveness can be understood in the following terms:

'the extent to which specific clinical interventions, when deployed in the field for a particular individual, group or population, do what they are intended to do. i.e. Maintain and improve health and secure the greatest possible health gain from the available resources. An intervention must be both clinically effective and cost effective and be shown to produce those benefits in practice.' (Chambers, 1998)

A King's Fund programme, Promoting Action on Clinical Effectiveness (PACE), is developing evidence-based practice as a routine way of working for health services. It has described the successful outcomes when clinical effectiveness is linked to local needs and priorities as long as clinicians, managers, policy makers and patients are all involved in the process (Chambers, 1998).

Consideration must also be taken of the cost-effectiveness of decision-making, 'to maximise the benefit to patients, given the constraints of scarce resources' (Pettite, 1994). Cost is now a part of every treatment decision and cost-effective decision-making is part of the rationing debate. There is a paradox here in that cost-effectiveness is concerned with relative benefits for populations of patients, while evidence-based practice is concerned with absolute benefit to the individual.

Audit forms the last stage in the process. Clinical audit helps the team reach a standard of working as close to best practice as possible.

Evidence-based practice and CAMHS

How 'evidence' is defined has major implications for the provision of CAMHS. A narrow view, for example that only randomised controlled trials (RCTs) should be considered when planning treatment interventions, may suit surgical and perhaps medical teams; however, RCTs are likely to have only a limited role in helping child mental health workers make decisions about interventions for young people. There are three principal reasons for this (Graham, 2000):

- Systemic thinking often considers the young person's symptoms as secondary to, or in the context of, a predicament they are experiencing. RCTs focus on comparing groups of individuals who have the same symptom cluster (diagnosis) and usually ignore their predicaments. It makes little sense to focus on symptoms and make no reference to context when the symptoms are clearly secondary and would often resolve spontaneously if the predicament were attended to.
- Ninety-five per cent of children attending CAMHS have more than one diagnosis (Audit Commission, 1999), yet the majority of RCTs are done to establish an intervention to improve the outcome of a single disorder. The presence of comorbidity is likely significantly to affect both intervention and likely outcome for the young person.
- Criteria for entry into the majority of RCTs generally demand that the subjects meet either ICD–10 or DSM research criteria for diagnosis of the disorder under study. Yet many young people who are suffering, and in need of help from CAMHS, do not achieve this level of diagnosis. Therefore the degree to which the results of the RCT are generalisable to this clinical population is doubtful.

It is important to recognise that different disorders respond to different therapies (Graham, 2000). Therefore CAMHS require members with expertise in behavioural therapy, cognitive–behavioural therapy, family therapy, individual psychodynamic psychotherapy and group therapy. Any gap in available skills will prevent the team practising in an evidence-based way when faced with a clinical problem for which evidence of efficacy for a specific therapy exists.

In general, when either might be applied, the evidence for the effectiveness of behavioural therapies is greater than that for non-behavioural therapies (see Box 7.4). This may reflect, however, that more behavioural therapies have been evaluated (Graham, 2000). Clearly, unevaluated therapies cannot be considered ineffective. The evidence for interventions in child and adolescent mental health has been recently reviewed (Fonagy *et al*, 2002; Wolpert *et al*, 2002).

Issues in practice

Treatment

How does any member of CAMHS decide whom to treat? Should an asthmatic child take precedence when there is a good evidence base that family therapy will reduce the incidence and severity of asthma attacks (Lask & Matthew, 1979) but the child has a low level of emotional disturbance? Or should work be directed to a conduct-disordered adolescent in the care of the local authority who will have massive psychological disturbance, but for whom there is no recognised curative intervention? The practice of evidence-based medicine dictates the former, but the need to support other agencies working with very difficult young people dictates the latter. A CAMHS therefore has to think very carefully about how it prioritises its workload and to have clear operational policies stating why it has those priorities, so that other agencies, professionals and management structures understand them.

Prevention

How do CAMHS professionals influence risk factors such as poverty, learning disability or bullying for the development of conditions when those risk factors are in operation before any referral and are often impervious to CAMHS intervention?

Professionals working in CAMHS are mainly involved in secondary and tertiary prevention through their clinical work. However, they may also be involved in primary prevention either through seeking to influence government policy (in education, employment policy, etc.) or local policy (e.g. housing), but these are political activities not defined by the professional role. CAMHS professionals may be involved in teaching or training outside the team with other agencies, whether statutory (e.g. social services, education), voluntary or academic (e.g.

Box 7.4 Evidence in child and adolescent mental health (after Graham, 2000)

Medication reduces symptoms in:
- attention deficit hyperactivity disorder (Weiss, 1996)
- psychotic disorders (McClellan & Werry, 1994)
- obsessive–compulsive disorders (DeVaugh-Geiss et al, 1992)
- Gilles de la Tourette's syndrome (Shapiro et al, 1989)
- enuresis, on a short-term basis (Blackwell & Currah, 1973)
- depression (Elmslie et al, 1997)

Cognitive–behavioural therapy is effective in:
- obsessive–compulsive disorders (March, 1995)
- bulimia in older adolescents (Wilson et al, 1991)
- generalised anxiety disorders and some phobias (Kendall & Southam-Gerow, 1996)
- post-traumatic stress disorder (Smith et al, 1998)
- depressive disorders (Harrington, 1998)
- non-organic pain disorders (Sanders et al, 1994)
- the enhancement of social skills (Beelman et al, 1994)
- the psychiatric consequences of sexual abuse (Jones & Ramchandani, 1999)

Other treatments:
- Family therapy is better than routine support and weight maintenance in adolescents with anorexia nervosa (Russell et al, 1987) and in the management of some medical problems associated with psychological symptoms (e.g. asthma) (Lask & Matthew, 1979).
- Psychoanalytic psychotherapy has been shown to improve compliance in difficult-to-control diabetes (Moran et al, 1991).
- Interpersonal therapy is promising in the treatment of adolescent depression (Fombonne, 1998).
- Behavioural therapies are useful in the treatment of enuresis (Dische et al, 1983).
- Parent management training reduces conduct disorder in young boys (Kazdin et al, 1992).
- Family therapy (Henggeler et al, 1998) and parent management training and family therapy (Kazdin, 1997) improve conduct disorder and reduce subsequent delinquency in older children of both genders (Kazdin, 1997).

university) or on an ad hoc basis as a result of local requests from statutory organisations or self-help groups. All of these heighten awareness of mental health issues and psychiatric disorders.

More directly, CAMHS professionals may provide consultation to a range of Tier 1 professionals who are seeing young people at risk of developing mental illness. In addition, they may develop, or be part of, multi-disciplinary groups arranging early intervention programmes for vulnerable children, such as an 'early bird' early intervention programme in pre-school autistic children or early intervention programmes for children at risk of conduct disorder (Little & Mount, 1999).

Outcomes

To whom are CAMHS professionals answerable in terms of the outcomes of their work – the children, their mothers, their fathers, their schools, their neighbours, their social workers, the police or the courts? They will all have their own expectations and it is unlikely they will all be the same. The welfare principle, subsequently known as the paramountcy principle, puts the child at the head of a CAMHS priority list. However, CAMHS have to work with the parents in most cases, so it is important not to alienate them. This is also true of schools, but CAMHS are not answerable to them. Only when considerations of abuse arise do responsibilities to the child through other agencies override those of the parents. CAMHS are required to work with other agencies but cannot let them dictate what should be the outcome of their work, or CAMHS become primarily agents of state control.

Conclusion

Evidence-based health care should aid team working by providing a common framework for problem solving and understanding between team members with different professional backgrounds. It may also contribute to removing hierarchical distinctions that are based on seniority, as any member of the team can perform a search and critical appraisal and then be in a position to advise others.

CHAPTER 8

User participation – participatory appraisal

Caroline Keir, Janet Harris and Barbara Webb

'Not everything that counts can be counted and not everything that can be counted counts'.
Albert Einstein

User participation

'User involvement' has become an increasingly significant theme in National Health Service (NHS) policy over recent years. Throughout the 1990s, Department of Health strategy documents advocated a more active and informed role for service users. In 1995, the NHS *Priorities and Planning Guidance* sought to give:

'greater voice and influence to users of NHS services and their carers in their own care, the development and definition of standards set for NHS services locally and the development of NHS policy both locally and nationally.' (NHS Executive, 1995)

As with many top-down initiatives, the influence of this rhetoric on grass-roots practice has been variable, resulting in pockets of good practice rather than a consistent national strategy.

Consumer organisations (e.g. the College of Health) and various research bodies have offered guidance on developing effective strategies for NHS service user involvement (Kelson, 1997). In general, they advocate active rather than passive involvement; service users should be allowed to set the agenda for change as well as to provide feedback in the context of service evaluation. Goss & Miller (1995), in their review of user involvement initiatives in community care, argue that there is a tendency in this work to place the 'organisations rather than user and carer needs at the centre of all thinking'. This recognition must be at the heart of user involvement in CAMHS.

Actively involving service users in service evaluation and development is a new concept in the NHS. In the past, clinicians have relied largely on questionnaires and patient satisfaction surveys to keep them up to date with how service users felt about the services they provided. However, when responding to a questionnaire, service users do not have a say in what questions should be asked, and cannot therefore raise issues that are not already on the agenda. In this sense their role is passive. The use of discussion groups or focus groups to elicit feedback allows more interaction between service users and service providers. Developing this process further requires service users to have an equal voice with service providers. Despite helpful guidelines on how to achieve equal standing, the waters are relatively uncharted.

Groups identified as potential participants in a user involvement project include the young people using the service, their families and close friends, the staff who provide the service, local voluntary organisations and other professionals who support or have contact with young people with mental health problems. The perspective of a range of young people, not just those who use the service, is also helpful.

The involvement of users has two distinct aims. The first is to help staff develop and negotiate patient-defined standards for the care of young people with mental health problems. The second is to ensure that all those involved understand from the outset that their contribution is both necessary and valuable, and that the intention is to make improvements to the service in line with the evaluation findings. Users are naturally suspicious of involvement that may turn out to be an 'empty' consultation exercise, with little to see from the results.

An evaluation or appraisal carried out by an external organisation is more likely to win the confidence of both users and providers. Fears that confidentiality and objectivity may be compromised by an evaluation being carried out by those within the organisation are serious considerations and provide a strong argument in favour of engaging external researchers. In addition, neutral outsiders are able to bring a fresh perspective that looks beyond organisational boundaries.

Participatory appraisal

Participatory appraisal is not the only evaluation method that can be used but it is a technique particularly appropriate to this client group. Young people generally are not known for their overwhelming willingness to be questioned about their personal lives by enquiring adults, and providing feedback about mental health services they have used (and may need to use again) is a subject upon which they may be expected to be reticent. A detailed description of participatory appraisal is described elsewhere (Chambers, 1994a,b; Rifkin et al, 2000). However, there are three key elements of participatory appraisal that indicate why it is especially suited to CAMHS:

- It advocates a 'whole community approach', where all those with a potential interest in the issue are invited to participate (further details from the authors on request). This approach aims to capture diverse opinions to ensure that all service needs and opinions are identified.

- It uses a wide range of interactive tools, such as mapping, ranking, listing, sorting, diagramming, timelines, causal impact analysis, brainstorming, semi-structured interviews and formal and informal group meetings. Participants select the most appropriate tools for sharing information, thereby increasing their ownership of the process. The tools generate a wide range of information that can be used for service planning (Cornwall & Jewkes, 1995).
- It has proven to be an effective technique for use with young people where winning their trust is vital to the research process (Harris *et al*, 2001).

Participatory appraisal is usually based on formal or informal group discussions, but in the context of CAMHS one-to-one work may be less threatening to service users. Initially, informal routes are used to try to make contact with young people. Voluntary organisations can be contacted, like MIND, and other local organisations with established links with young people. The service provider may seek permission from service users to pass on their contact details to the project facilitator or they may act as intermediaries, writing to the young people and inviting them to contact the facilitators directly. In either case, potential participants can be assured that the service provider will not know who has been accepted to participate in the project. Letters sent inviting young people to participate should give assurances that their contribution will be anonymous and that their confidentiality will be respected.

Trained facilitators conduct one-to-one sessions. It may be helpful to put the sessions on a more equal footing by having the participants choose the location for the meeting, as they may choose to meet in their home, or at a familiar setting such as a local café. During the sessions, participants use timelines, mapping, ranking and force field analysis to describe their views of the CAMHS. Sessions should last about two hours. After the individual sessions, some participants may agree to participate in follow-up group sessions.

Having a mental health problem is a traumatic experience for a young person and family. Many participants find it difficult to talk about their experiences, particularly at the start of the session. However, those who are involved in group work seem to enjoy the opportunity to meet, reminisce about experiences and reflect on what has happened to them.

The young people are, of course, the primary participants, but they are asked to pass on information about the project to anyone else they think might be able to contribute. In this way contact may be made with parents and siblings.

Group work with service staff should be organised through the team with overall responsibility for the service.

As is usual in projects of this sort, participants need to be offered back-up counselling support if desired and facilitators should also have debriefing support. This helps the facilitator to avoid falling into a pseudo-counselling role.

Throughout the project, care must be taken to represent accurately the information that is offered by participants. One-to-one interviews and group work are summarised and given to participants for verification. All those who have participated in the study are also encouraged to comment on a draft report to ensure that their views have been accurately represented. Following the production of a final report it is important to set up some mechanism (e.g. a steering group) both to identify an action plan and to oversee its implementation.

Key learning points

This section draws on the authors' experiences across a range of projects, to demystify the process of involving service users.

Ensuring diversity: identifying and contacting people

If the aim is to involve young people, they should be written to directly. In this way they receive the same courtesy as an adult, and are allowed control over whether they participate or not. Where children are under 16, the parent or guardian must be informed of the invitation to participate. However, they can be informed in a separate letter, thereby preserving direct contact with the young person.

The objectivity and confidentiality of the process are important. Service users are often reluctant to become involved if they think that their comments will be made known to staff who have been, or might become, involved in their care. It is important to emphasise that the facilitators have no direct involvement with the CAMHS.

In any sort of evaluation that involves service users, it is important to be patient. Word of mouth usually brings forward more respondents and the project will generate its own momentum. Several attempts may be needed over 12 months to elicit a good initial response. If contact is continued, it is likely that more respondents will come forward.

An appropriately stratified sample is ideal, but in the end the exercise depends on who responds. However, it is very important to be clear about those who have not been included, as well as those who have, and highlight the implications of this. This may give an imbalance in the service user perspective, but it is better than no service user perspective at all, which allows organisational concerns to assume priority.

Empowerment and ownership of the process

The implication of empowering service users is that their perspective is as important as other perspectives, including that of staff. Ideally, while not controlling the process, staff should have a sense of ownership as joint stakeholders. Ownership, however, can be compromised if the project facilitators are outsiders, as well as by staff attitudes towards ownership.

In some settings, projects may have to function within existing hierarchies, which will allow staff to voice their views but may limit their ownership of the project. It is essential that senior managers (i.e. those who control resources) are committed to the project and to the principle of service user involvement, and that they have confidence in the process and will act upon the findings. Without this, the time and resources of both staff and service users are being wasted.

Documenting and managing the process: building trust among participants

Participants should be kept in touch with the project at key stages. Ideally, a representative from all participating groups should be included in a steering group to take the work forward.

It takes courage for service providers to listen to feedback and they need to be reassured that there will be benefits. In this context, the presentation of findings is crucial. Reports should provide a balanced account of participants' perspectives. Discussions of findings should encourage staff to celebrate the positive before moving on to the more sensitive issues that service users raise.

A principal concern among staff is that service users will be too demanding. However, there is usually a good deal of common ground between the concerns of staff and the concerns of service users. Williamson (1992) refers to this common ground as 'synergistic interests'. She suggests that 'deep feelings direct the hope in us all that synergistic interests will be common and non-synergistic rare'. The common ground certainly provides the potential to make positive change and develop greater trust between participants. A useful role for external advisors on the project would be to ensure that non-synergistic issues are not overlooked.

Service users are often very pragmatic; they are sympathetic to resource issues and other difficulties that confront staff and they can often help staff find solutions that do not involve extra resources. Service users themselves can be used as a resource. In the context of adult mental health services, service users have contributed to staff training, written information leaflets for in-patients and drafted job descriptions for nursing assistants and standards for ward rounds.

Conclusion

This chapter has provided guidance on how to involve users in the evaluation of services. If the service is provided in a multi-agency environment, then a 'whole community approach' to service user involvement is particularly apposite. Through the involvement of the voluntary sector and local authority youth workers, organisational boundaries may be crossed. Service users are often enthusiastic about having been given a voice that would not otherwise have been heard. A number remain keen to keep in touch and some even welcome more active involvement. It is important that, in the process of empowering service users, staff do not feel disempowered; getting this balance right is difficult. Effective participation is likely if:

- repeated attempts are made to find many different kinds of participants
- approaches that allow participants some control over the process (in terms of meeting times and tools) are used
- participants are facilitated in the voicing of diverse points of view
- stakeholders (such as service providers) are actively involved, to ensure that user involvement is seen as a valuable commodity
- a 'no surprises' approach to the findings is ensured, by sharing viewpoints and findings throughout the course of the project.

CHAPTER 9

Training

Nick Jones, Ian Partridge and Barry Wright

EDUCATION, n. That which discloses to the wise and disguises from the foolish their lack of understanding.
Ambrose Bierce

Introduction

Increased medical advances, and challenges posed by a better-informed and more demanding public, have put pressure on clinicians both to perform and to show themselves to perform at higher standards than ever before. National standards have been set through National Service Frameworks (NSFs) and through the National Institute for Clinical Excellence (NICE). Central to the setting, delivering and monitoring of these standards is clinical governance. Although professional self-regulation provides clinicians with the opportunity to help set standards, *A First Class Service* (Department of Health, 1998c) recognised that only lifelong learning would give staff in the National Health Service (NHS) the tools of knowledge to offer the most modern, effective and high-quality care to patients. In addition, it would allow the identification of training needs across all professions and thereby aid team working. Continuing professional development (CPD) has for a long time met the learning needs of individual professionals while inspiring public confidence in their skills as clinicians.

In order to meet the challenges of the new NHS, stronger links are required between CPD, audit, clinical effectiveness, and research and development. CAMHS therefore require health professionals, and their professional bodies, local employers, higher-education providers and local education consortia, to develop CPD programmes that meet both local service needs and those of the professional. A CAMHS is made up from a group of already qualified professionals who have undertaken extensive training in their own discipline. If it is to be truly multi-disciplinary and multi-agency, then it follows that any 'specialist' training should also be multi-disciplinary and joint-agency based.

Box 9.1 Components of a training strategy

- Local health improvement programme (HIMP).
- Identification of the needs of the local population.
- A CAMHS strategy.
- Inter-agency and multi-disciplinary working.
- Established operational policies.
- Individual post specifications.
- Individual development/appraisal reviews.

Educational strategy

The modern CAMHS should have an integrated multi-disciplinary education strategy based on the principles listed in Box 9.1.

All staff, irrespective of grade or profession, require personal development plans (PDPs) to ensure that they have a clear professional understanding of their individual skills and that they can master their role within the team. The result should be a training programme that meets agreed objectives. Annual development/appraisal reviews serve to recognise milestones, to offer feedback and to provide guidance and monitoring. Training should not be seen as a once and for all process but as a dynamic continuum and investment for the future. It must:

- be relevant and valued by the CAMHS
- enhance child, family and services
- be cost-effective
- be disseminated to other members of the service.

Learning climate and methods of training

Critten (1993) has described the conditions necessary for effective learning and suggests the establishment of a 'learning company' as an organisation able to create a climate in which individual members are encouraged to learn and to develop their full potential. Progressive CAMHS will create an atmosphere where learning and working are synonymous, promoting both collective and self-direction in order to meet the continuing process of care transformation. Training should be seen as cyclical, a continuous process of reviewing and developing care in light of evaluation. Peaks and troughs in training are a reaction to change, while continual training is instrumental to change.

Different forms of training (Box 9.2) all have worth, depending on individual need, and not all training or learning has to be formal. Many CAMHS members can benefit greatly from a period of approved 'time out', whereby time is allocated both to reflect upon and to investigate

---

Box 9.2 Types of training

- I do, you do, training.
- Coaching.
- Courses, seminars, workshops, conferences.
- Project work.
- Academic study.
- Time out/reading.
- Job rotation/exchange.

---

contemporary clinical practice. The creation of a library is a vital training tool, as is internet access to enable evidence-based practice to be found via the Cochrane Library, the NHS Centre for Review and Dissemination, electronic library for health and other useful websites. A regulated library system may also go some way to alleviating fears of absent books and pilfering. A commitment to team training and open learning can assist all, and helps to avoid the stockpiling of information and library books in service members' offices.

Multi-disciplinary training

All disciplines within a CAMHS will have undertaken professional training. Post-qualification 'specialist' training is usually undertaken, specific to working with young persons and their families, to develop skills and interests. Successful CAMHS will contain a strong element of inter-disciplinary working. The strength of this working lies in its access to a wide range of skills.

Yearly review/development plans and a service training needs analysis should reflect the need for joint training and be budgeted accordingly. There is often an inequity of training opportunities and training budgets within the CAMHS. A way of managing this is to agree a principle of service training needs and to prioritise them from the training budget. The pooling of training budgets can be a challenge for individual disciplines but is a positive step towards shared learning. Teams may need to be creative in their funding for training and may consider sponsorship or the creation of a 'slush' fund from the proceeds of team-facilitated study days or from teaching commitments to other organisations.

Inter-agency team training

Working Together (Department of Health, 1988) set the scene for the integration of health and social care and led to joint training agencies being established throughout the country, of which the National

Children's Bureau and the training centre of the National Society for the Prevention of Cruelty to Children, in Leicester, are two examples. *The Hybrid Worker* (John Brown, 1994) illustrated how shared learning between health and social care staff contributed to positive integrated care within learning disabilities services. *Our Healthier Nation* (Department of Health, 1998*b*) and *Children in Mind* (Audit Commission, 1999) pointed towards the joint commissioning of mental health services for children. In response to this many local CAMHS, in conjunction with other statutory agencies, produced multi-agency strategies and subsequent action plans for children's services. It appears logical that joint services should require joint training for the professionals involved. In many areas this has resulted in multi-agency CAMHS training strategies being established, with the intention of integrating training opportunities for staff across organisations. These initiatives have led to:

- the establishment of joint training on issues of common interest
- the development of a local register of training capacity and opportunities within each agency and open access to training across agencies
- liaison with neighbouring CAMHS training groups for regional training and audit
- liaison with carers' groups and voluntary agencies to extend training opportunities
- the establishment of joint training and courses with local educational institutions/universities.

CAMHS as providers of training

Child and adolescent mental health professionals have a role in providing training for Tier 1 services. This training may be in a formal setting, such as a workshop or seminar, but is just as likely to occur informally, through surgeries, consultations or direct clinical supervision. Whatever the venue, it is important the 'teacher' feels adequately prepared and skilled to teach the session. The training needs of the trainers should not be overlooked and opportunity should be given for trainers to practise and to be given structured feedback on their performance. This can be achieved by a system of mentoring by the more experienced members of staff and, if appropriate, by calling upon the expertise of the local university or higher-education departments for advice and support. In addition, if the team offers training regularly, they may consider producing a feedback/evaluation form for use at later supervision sessions.

Presentation skills are important, as successful teams are often invited to present their work at local or national conferences.

Links with further-education establishments

Clinical governance, the NSFs, NICE, health improvement and NHS research and development programmes are all making great demands upon clinicians. If these initiatives are to succeed within CAMHS, partnerships are demanded by the complexity and the sheer volume of work set before the services. One key partnership is the relationship between CAMHS and the local university or further-educational establishment. Local departments of health studies can play a vital role in providing training for all members of the CAMHS. For example, team teaching and the development of the nurse/therapist/practitioner role can enhance the quality of such courses as the ENB 603 Child and Adolescent Nursing Course and other discipline/group training (and provide a potential source of income for further training). In addition, social policy departments can provide vital links in the dissemination of information regarding national policy and trends. CAMHS should actively foster good working relationships with these departments in order both to underpin their practice and to support them in the pursuit of lifelong learning.

CHAPTER 10

Court work

Greg Richardson and Geraldine Casswell

> No man is exempt from saying silly things. The misfortune is to say them seriously.
> Michel Eyquem de Montaigne

Introduction

The child's welfare is the primary consideration when preparing a court report, no matter who has commissioned it or who will pay for it (Department of Health, 1991). This principle must be clear throughout any work for the courts, as the possibility of a specific opinion being paid for can bring the professions into disrepute. A structure for addressing court work is required. Advice is available for both clinical psychologists (British Psychological Society, 2000) and psychiatrists (Black *et al*, 1998; Tuffnell *et al*, 1996).

Questions to consider

Does the request come from a solicitor?

Requests for reports for the court must always come from a solicitor. Requests by parents, carers or social workers for court reports should be refused, or directed back to the solicitor. Requests not agreed by the court are likely to be viewed as partisan. There has been a move over recent years for joint instructions to be issued for expert opinion, in an attempt to lessen the adversarial nature of children's proceedings. Writing a report always involves a possibility of being called to court to justify it.

Does the report concern a young person with whom the professional is currently clinically involved?

Professional witnesses account for their work with a young person and family and explain any conclusions drawn from that work. Such witnesses may be referred to as a 'witness to fact', in that they are giving evidence as to the 'facts' of their involvement with the case. In

Table 10.1 Considerations for professional and expert witnesses writing in court reports

Professional witness	Expert witness
Confidentiality	Time
Effect of the report on the therapeutic relationship	Not primarily a therapeutic relationship
Effect of the therapeutic relationship on impartiality	Impartial
May charge for the report only if the assessment work is not undertaken as part of NHS duties	May charge for all preparatory work as well as the report

contrast, an expert witness comes new to the situation to assess what is in the child's best interests (see Table 10.1).

It is important to understand why a report is being requested and, if clinically involved, the effect preparing a report will have on the on-going therapeutic alliance.

Is it a civil or a criminal matter?

Civil matters are those where the court is trying to decide what is the best option for a child's future development. They arise when children have suffered significant harm (Adcock & White, 1998) or their welfare has become a secondary consideration of those responsible for their care, or where a child is seeking to claim compensation (e.g. after an accident or medical error). Children Act proceedings are generally civil matters, and the expert or professional witness is being asked what actions would be in the child's best interests (this can include issues of contact or issues of the granting of supervision or care orders). The new rules of civil procedure enshrine the general principle of the use of a single expert witnesses.

Criminal matters arise when the young person has committed an offence and the court wishes to know whether the young person is suffering from a mental illness or has some psychological difficulties that represent mitigating factors. Occasionally, but rarely, opinion may be sought in support of a 'not guilty' plea. It is helpful to be aware of the major reforms in youth justice and the establishment of youth justice teams resulting from the Crime and Disorder Act 1998.

It should be borne in mind that, when recommending treatment of any kind, the treatment is available and who will do it has been negotiated. Local CAMHS do not take kindly to being told by the courts what treatment they will undertake because of the recommendations of a distant expert who has taken the money and run; nor do the CAMHS have any obligation to take the work on.

Has the request for the report been agreed between all parties?

Increasingly, the courts do not wish to have conflicting evidence from expert witnesses, because of the extra expense and court time. It is therefore important to ensure that the solicitor commissioning a report is speaking on behalf of all parties involved in the case. If this is not checked, the professional may be seen as being in one party's camp (e.g. the father's witness), or become involved in the indelicacy of intra-professional confrontations in court.

What are the questions that require answers in the report?

In general, courts request reports for a purpose. They wish to ensure that all relevant matters are taken into consideration when making their decision and require answers to certain questions. It is important to understand the questions in order to address them. It may also be helpful to clarify questions that are beyond the professional's competence (e.g. the prognosis of an illness in a parent, when a child specialist may direct the solicitor to a more appropriate expert). The questions should be clearly laid out in the letter of instruction, and it should be established that the court has given leave to interview all relevant parties and read all relevant documentation; a professional witness may not have access to all the documentation. It is important to have expertise in the areas about which an opinion is being sought – for example, experience with adolescents with a learning disability or where there is dispute as to whether a child has been sexually abused (Jones, 1992). If in doubt, withdrawal at this stage is preferable to humiliation later, when ignorance is exposed.

What is the time-scale for the preparation of the report?

The Children Act 1989 quite rightly lays down that legal matters concerning children should be dealt with as expeditiously as possible (Department of Health, 1991), as children's development is always at risk while they are awaiting court decisions. It is therefore necessary to understand the court's expectations in terms of a report's preparation. If it is not possible to meet a deadline, it is important to say so and to determine a realistic time-scale. The time-scale must take account of the amount of documentation to be read and the number of interviews to be undertaken. It is better not to be pressured into underestimating the amount of time required. Once a deadline is agreed, it is important to meet it, for elaborate and expensive court processes will be planned around it. It is important to be aware that the pressures on the courts often generate unreasonable expectations in terms of how quickly reports can be prepared.

Table 10.2 Terms of address in court

Type of court	Terms of address
Magistrates	Sir, Ma'am, Your Worship
County and Crown Court judges	Your Honour
High Court judges	My Lord, My Lady, Your Lordship, Your Ladyship

In which court is the case being heard?

It is helpful to know the level of the court that is requesting the report, as this will influence how much background and explanation the report will require. For example, magistrates may not have as sophisticated an understanding of child development and the roles of CAMHS professionals as will a High Court judge. Also, the terms of address differ between courts (Table 10.2).

Magistrates' courts are local, county courts are in the nearest large town and High Court sittings are only in large cities. Magistrates' courts deal with juvenile offenders and the 'family panel' with some Children Act issues. County courts deal with Children Act cases passed to them by the magistrates because of their complexity, so a report prepared for the magistrates' court may be passed to the county court. The Crown Court hears appeals from Children Act proceedings and deals with some juvenile offenders. The Family Division of the High Court deals with contested Children Act proceedings, contested adoptions and with 'wardship', which has become far less common since the introduction of the Children Act 1989. Children Act cases are dealt with at family centres, in which the case is heard 'in chambers', which means the public and press do not have access and the legal professionals do not wear full regalia. Appeals against judgements in these courts go to the Court of Appeal and then the House of Lords (Mitchels & Meadows, 1989; Williams, 1992).

Charging for the report

The solicitor may forget to ask, so it is important to inform him or her of the charges the preparation of a report will incur. Differential rates for preparation work, interviews, travel, and court appearances and so on may be appropriate. It is not reasonable to charge for clinical work undertaken as part of NHS commitments if the information is subsequently used in the preparation of a report. However, it is reasonable to charge for the time involved in the preparation of the report, because this would not normally be part of clinical care and extra work is involved in the preparation of the report.

How much to charge is probably best discussed with colleagues. If the child and family are in receipt of legal aid, the solicitor should ask for a written estimate of fees and expenses so that he or she can submit a claim to the Legal Aid Board. If this is not done, there is no assurance that the fees will be paid.

Until the implementation of the new consultant contract, medical members of CAMHS have a curious anomaly that sets them apart from other members of the team. They are entitled to do category 2 work, for which fees may be charged, but which does not count as private practice. In essence, all legal work is categorised as category 2. This raises ethical issues for doctors regarding how much of their time they can devote to legal work. If they take on category 2 work during their normal working hours, they are being paid twice and may be at risk of neglecting patients with other needs. Using half days and/or weekends may resolve this dilemma. For non-medical members of CAMHS, the issue is much simpler: if they prepare reports on young people or families who are not their patients, this is private work and cannot be undertaken as part of their NHS duties. If they know the patient, they may prepare a report and attend court within working hours and may charge for this.

It is important to submit an account of charges, which should be detailed, with the report. Most solicitors will pay the account within a reasonable length of time, although they may first have to submit it to the Legal Aid Board. Occasionally rogue solicitors are reluctant to settle their accounts, so it is sometimes wise to request payment after the report is prepared but before it is submitted.

Whom to see and what to read

Whom to see and what to read will be determined by the content of the report; seeing people and reading give information on the child's development so far, and so provide the platform on which the assessment and opinion of what is in the child's best interests is based.

In preparing a professional report, on someone seen clinically, most of the information for the report should be in the file. However, if working with a mother and child, to prepare a comprehensive report, it may be necessary to see an estranged father. Before doing so, it is important to seek clarification as to issues of parental responsibility and residence. Setting up appointments with family members who have not been involved in treatment can be problematic. An uninvolved expert does not have these problems; this may explain why more guardians are now requesting expert opinions and generally prefer these to those of local services (Brophy et al, 1999).

In coming to the case without previous contact, it is useful to discuss with the commissioning solicitor who they think should be seen. A guardian may have been appointed and a discussion with guardians may be helpful as they will have a detailed knowledge of the case and will be able to identify the salient people. Sometimes it is less disruptive to see children in their own home, but awareness of physical and professional safety may necessitate taking a colleague. In residence and contact disputes it is necessary to see both parents, and in issues involving the local authority it is necessary to talk to the social worker and possibly foster parents or residential care workers. In compensation cases it is not usually necessary to interview the perpetrator of the accident but copies of the medical notes will be essential for claims of medical negligence.

It is reasonable to ask solicitors to obtain documents that may be helpful in the preparation of the report. Supporting statements by involved parties, case conference minutes and school reports are basic essentials, but other documentation, such as previous medical records, may also be required to reach an informed view.

Preparation of the report

There are published guidelines on how to write a legal report (Black *et al*, 1998), the format proposed by Tuffnell (1993) being recommended at the time by the Official Solicitor to the Supreme Court. The work of the Official Solicitor has now been incorporated into the Children and Family Court Advisory Support Service (CAFCASS). *The Expert Witness Pack* (Vizard & Harris, 1997) is also a great help.

The front of the report should contain the name of the child and date of birth, the nature of the proceedings, the court reference number/s, the name, qualifications and working address of the person preparing the report, the date of the report and a table of contents. The subsequent sections are outlined in Table 10.3.

The report should be written on A4 paper in a font size of at least 12 point, double-spaced and with wide margins. Sections and paragraphs should be numbered, as should the pages. The report should be written in short, uncomplicated sentences; jargon and technical terminology should be avoided, as should overcomplicated or ambiguous argument. Succinct reports that are to the point are appreciated. They allow the giving of evidence in a clear fashion.

Appearing in court

Most requests for a court report do not result in a court appearance. If the professional is to appear, the date should be established as soon as possible, as the court appearance will disrupt clinical schedules. Some hearings are listed for several days, so it is perfectly reasonable to state availability, after discussion and agreement with the commissioning

Table 10.3 Format for court reports

Section	Content
Introduction	The introduction should cover who has asked for the report to be prepared, the nature of the proceedings, the reasons for the preparation of the report and the questions the report has to address. Sources of information and relevant curriculum vitae should be referred to as appendices.
Background	This section should contain a chronological listing of relevant facts in the development of the child and any background literature or knowledge base that is referred to.
Assessment	The assessment section should contain views, opinions and deductions from the background information. It is often helpful to include a consideration of the Welfare Checklist (Williams, 1992) to clarify to the court that matters identified as important in the Children Act 1989 have been considered. The report is geared to stating what is in the best interests of the child; however, by the time of the report the best interests of the child have often been damaged by that child's life experience. It is the report writer's task to determine which is the least detrimental option for the child's future and to describe how that option might be enhanced for the child's benefit.
Opinion	This section contains conclusions from the assessment section and is where the questions detailed in the introduction are addressed.
Recommendation	The recommendation section states clearly what action is necessary to ensure the best interests of the child. A report prepared in a compensation case may well not have any recommendations, as it is opinion that is required.
Conclusion	Conclude with the sentence 'I believe that the facts I have stated in this report are true and that the opinions I have expressed are correct' (recommendation by Jordans Solicitors, 1999, personal communication) and sign the report.
Appendices	Appendices should detail who has been interviewed and what documents were considered in the preparation of the report. Separate appendices may cover the details of specific interviews, and curriculum vitae. In civil cases a copy of the letter of instruction should be appended.

solicitor. Courts do keep professional and expert witnesses waiting for lengths of time that would not be acceptable for families in clinics. Court hearings often occur some considerable time after the report has been submitted and a lot of clinical material will have flowed under the practice bridge between the two events. It is therefore imperative to read the report and re-establish the salient background factors that led to the conclusions. It is sensible to ask the instructing solicitor to forward any relevant new documents, should they become available.

On the day of the court appearance the 'court suit' should be clean and pressed – for some reason courts consider that impeccable opinions come only from the impeccably dressed. It is also a display of respect to those involved in the hearing, as well as the court itself. Plenty of time should be allowed to get to the court – ensure arrival in good time. It is a good idea to know which judge is sitting, as court listings will then establish the location of the hearing.

Occasionally professional or expert witnesses may be asked to see members of the family or another professional to clarify issues of possible contention. Generally it is worthwhile agreeing with this, as it removes adversarial discussions from the courtroom and means the court can devote its time to deciding on the best interests of the child rather than which of differing opinions they are going to act upon. Such discussions may result in not having to give evidence at all.

When called upon to give evidence, after taking the oath, the solicitor or barrister will lead the witness through the 'evidence in chief'. This is the easy bit and all that is necessary is to watch the judge and ensure he or she has finished writing before continuing giving evidence. Cross-examination can give cause for concern, so marshalling experience and knowledge in relation to the case is of supreme importance (Reder *et al*, 1994). Competent witnesses never make a statement beyond their expertise, and never become angry or determined to win the point. Occasionally, taking a metaphorical step back and remembering the game-like qualities of the situation can offer an oasis of calm for the witness. This may seem to undermine the gravitas of the situation, but the child whose interests are being represented will be far better served by a thoughtful, measured presentation than an emotionally unpredictable, reactive diatribe (Wolkind, 1994). Tactics that facilitate taking a step back include sipping from a glass of water, asking for the question to be repeated or addressing the bench for clarification. In all cases answers should be addressed to the bench rather than the examining solicitor or barrister.

When evidence is completed, the barrister or solicitor will usually request that the witness be given leave to go.

Training issues

To increase the interest, knowledge and confidence of CAMHS professionals in undertaking court work affecting children and young people, it may be helpful for them all to do the following:

- prepare a report for a child protection case conference
- attend at least one child protection case conference per year
- prepare a report for a statutory agency or the courts on a case with which they are involved

---

Box 10.1 Training needs for court work

- To have a working knowledge of the legal frameworks affecting children and young people.
- To know how to plan and undertake assessments for statutory authorities and the courts.
- To have experience in preparing and writing court reports in an effective and acceptable way.
- To develop confidence in courtroom skills.
- To develop knowledge of how to access more detailed information on legal issues relating to children and young people.
- To clarify understanding of legal instructions.
- To plan and undertake assessments in both civil and criminal cases.
- To develop a functional and understandable format for court reports.
- To use a knowledge base in legal proceedings.
- To develop the capacity to represent children and their needs by understanding the paramountcy principle, especially in an adversarial legal process.
- To understand court structures and processes.
- To understand the Welfare Checklist and use it in the interests of the child.

- visit a court hearing to watch an experienced witness
- attend a workshop on writing reports for court and courtroom skills
- work with colleagues from other disciplines to prepare a report on a child at risk
- spend some time in joint work with a member of a youth offending team.

Court work can be stressful. There is a hierarchy of regard present in how courts hear from different disciplines and this, along with the fact that the legal world is different to the clinical world, means that training is imperative. Court can be a minefield for the uninitiated and the unprepared. Box 10.1 lists the training needs for court work.

CHAPTER 11

Strategies for moving into Tier 1

Greg Richardson and Ian Partridge

'Where men are not acquainted with each other's principles, nor experienced in each other's talents, nor at all practised in their mutual habitudes and disputations by joint efforts in business; no personal confidence, no friendship, no common interest, subsisting among them; it is evidently impossible that they can act a public part with uniformity, perseverance or efficacy.'
Edmund Burke, *Selections from the Speeches and Writings*

Introduction

Mental health problems in children are best understood as being affected by, and presenting in, the children's constitutional functioning and in all areas of their interaction with their environment. Parents, families and teachers have the major role to play in the maintenance of mental health. Professionals such as childminders, teachers, school nurses, educational psychologists, social workers, general practitioners and health visitors make a substantial contribution to the promotion and maintenance of the mental health of children. They also play a role in the early identification of mental health problems, children's vulnerability thereto and in the management of them once identified.

Mental health professionals, who provide a small part of the mental health care of children, classify the more serious mental health problems as mental disorders (World Health Organization, 1992). These disorders represent a small proportion of mental health problems produced by constitutional factors, family, educational, social and environmental difficulty, illness or developmental delay, all of which may impair future psychological functioning. More severe disorders, such as pervasive developmental disorders, tend to be managed largely by educational interventions, with psychological components such as behaviour modification rather than medical intervention.

Referral

There is a tendency for Tier 1 workers to seek referral of children to specialist agencies when they develop a concern regarding mental health problems. The tendency arises because they undervalue both their own relationships with the families and their abilities in the management of the difficulties being presented. The problem of Tier 1 professionals feeling deskilled or disempowered is one for which CAMHS professionals must take a degree of responsibility. A common understanding of terms such as 'mental health problems' and their integration with the language of other disciplines is required if children are not to suffer, as each agency defines problematic children in terms that give the responsibility for their management to others.

Mental health is an issue for all agencies who deal with children. The need for, and the problems with, the integration of agencies' working have been eloquently discussed from 'a clear educational perspective' (Dessent, 1996). Without accessible support and a shared language, the needs of the individual child can get lost in the process of institutional dialogue and discord. This will produce a fragmented and compartmentalised approach to mental health, and the application of a simplistic model of linear causality and problem solving, in which children's mental health problems can be seen and 'treated' in a vacuum, by specialists offering a 'cure'. Child mental health should not be regarded as a curative science but rather as offering more or less helpful advice and management in liaison with those involved with the developing child, be they parents or other professionals.

These are complex and emotionally difficult issues, which must be confronted if children's mental health problems are to be addressed in the situations in which they arise; it is inappropriate to assume that referral to CAMHS will solve all problems. Traditional 'medical' referral pathways provide security for those bewildered and made anxious by the children, young people and families with whom they have to deal. Ultimately, the only reason that referrals are made to a CAMHS is the existence of anxiety on somebody's part – be it the child, family or professional – and the belief that 'something must be done'. It is also true that people working with children and young people at Tier 1 are generally dissatisfied with CAMHS (NHS Health Advisory Service, 1995b; Audit Commission, 1999) and do not consider their needs are being met. Those trying to break down institutionalised referral pathways often find themselves at the receiving end of Tier 1 professionals' frustrations, and are perceived as instituting blocking strategies and failing to meet the legitimate needs of their clients.

The Audit Commission review of CAMHS in England and Wales (Audit Commission, 1999) demonstrated that child and adolescent mental health professionals spend only 1% of their time supporting Tier 1. As 90% of children and young people with a recognisable mental health problem are never seen by CAMHS, this is worrying. The study also showed that where primary mental health workers are in place referrals to Tiers 2, 3 and 4 are reduced.

If parents are asked how they would feel if their child was referred to a CAMHS, the feelings of being blamed, stigmatised, incompetent, bewildered and frightened often outweigh those of relief or feeling the problem is being taken seriously. Their mental health and self-esteem can thereby be seen to have been seriously assaulted by the referral process, even if it was poor prior to referral, even though, generally, mental health professionals are aware of the vulnerability of referred families. The input of Tier 1 professionals may therefore be considerably more helpful to the mental health of a young person and family than referral into Tier 2.

Tier 1 professionals are those who, by virtue of their job, have regular daily contact with children and, indeed, can have a profound effect on children's psychological development. A first filter separates children, young people and their families from this tier of professionals who work directly with children and therefore impinge to a greater or lesser extent on their mental health in the normal course of the children's lives. These professionals in turn operate a second filter, by deciding when it is necessary to involve professionals from Tier 2.

Moving into Tier 1 is therefore the major priority for CAMHS if they are to lay any claim to meeting the needs of the majority of young people with mental health problems and to do effective preventive work. Moving into Tier 1 requires considerable thought and planning. The expectations, understandings, beliefs and sophistication of those working at Tier 1 are varied. Basic lessons about 'incurability', allied to the need for management of certain disorders to be the responsibility of all involved in the care of young people, need to be owned and understood by all those working at Tier 1 to avoid unrealistic demands and expectations.

Support for Tier 1

Support for Tier 1 professionals should arise from their development of a relationship with a locally based CAMHS or person whom they can use for advice, consultation and as an information source. Such locality multi-agency working should ensure that Tier 1 professionals, as well as parents, carers and children, are supported and given confidence in their coping. Such mental health promotion can reduce referral to CAMHS.

Tier 1 work should result in the involvement of users in the planning and provision of CAMHS; families can also have an indirect input into the service and how it is provided. Inter-agency Tier 1 work can encourage inter-agency training and integrated case management through inter-agency assessment and review procedures.

Initiatives in Tier 1 working

A role for a primary mental health worker was suggested in *Together We Stand* (NHS Health Advisory Service, 1995a); this worker is a professional from CAMHS who develops relationships in a particular locality and empowers Tier 1 professionals in their work with the mental health of children. This has been put into practice in Portsmouth, where the establishment of such a post:

- identified unmet need
- decreased referrals to the CAMHS
- improved the quality of referrals to the CAMHS
- increased levels of satisfaction among Tier 1 professionals with the CAMHS
- developed inter-agency working and led to other inter-agency initiatives such as the joint school and family support team.

Having had a pilot primary mental health worker serving eight general practices, they now deploy eight primary mental health workers, drawn from psychologists and community psychiatric nurses, for a population of 600 000. These findings are now being replicated elsewhere.

The concept of the community mental health worker was developed in South Tees (Wilson & Waters, 1997); a person was employed to 'achieve better communication and develop networks with primary care staff'. This opening of communication channels enabled:

- referrals to the CAMHS to be more appropriate
- the discussion of potential referrals by Tier 1 workers with the community mental health worker
- Tier 1 staff to understand the work undertaken by the CAMHS
- the effective prioritisation of cases through community knowledge
- referrers to be kept in contact with the progress made by families who were involved with CAMHS
- families to feel more informed about what was happening to them.

Tier 1 specialisation recognises that certain staff, such as health visitors and school nurses, already perform a considerable amount of mental health work and with appropriate supplementary training and supervision could take on work that might otherwise be referred to CAMHS. Such development work has been undertaken in Northern Ireland, where educational programmes have been provided for health visitors by a member of the CAMHS (further details available from G.R. on request), so that they felt better equipped to deal with the mental health issues with which they are faced every day of their working lives. School nurses and health visitors find they are dealing with children's psychological problems but often consider themselves ill trained to do so. Training and consultation allow them to fulfil that function more effectively and confidently; these workers may then feel able to provide a within-school or surgery service (Richardson & Partridge, 2000). However, there still remain stigmatisation issues for children who choose to go to see these professionals, especially if they are known to have taken on this mental health role.

Consultation services in primary care (Garralda, 1994) and in non-medical settings have been used for many years (Nicol, 1994) as well as in residential settings (Silveira, 1991). However, they often seem unappreciated by those devoted to the referral system. In order to coordinate community services and prevent stigmatising referral to mental health services, it may be possible, especially with the advent of primary mental health workers providing consultation services, to reach a stage whereby there is no referral into CAMHS without prior consultation. This will ensure interventions at the Tier 1 level can be suggested and the concerns of the referrer discussed and addressed.

The Royal College of Psychiatrists and patient support groups publish management guidelines for a range of conditions. Information is also available on the internet, but this is often conflicting and variable in quality. Local CAMHS may therefore consider it worthwhile to publish guidelines on the management of common mental health problems for Tier 1 professionals, as well as letting them know the sorts of problems for which there are effective interventions.

Considerable liaison work needs to be done at Tier 1 to prevent these initiatives merely becoming elaborate referral routes into CAMHS, but if successfully achieved it may move Tier 1 support to the forefront of CAMHS.

Objectives of a primary mental health worker

A primary mental health worker would have the following objectives:

- to ensure that all who work directly with children and families have access to information about mental health services, advice, support and training for the mental health aspects of that role
- to ensure that professionals who support children and families – from statutory and non-statutory agencies – work closely together in a coordinated way, to ensure greater benefit for those receiving services (this can be achieved through multi-agency assessment of need, case management, multi-agency information systems, cross-agency supervision and joint study days or exchanges)
- to ensure young people and families within the locality are fully aware of the support and services available to them (e.g. by collecting information on local services and ensuring it is readily available in schools)

- to ensure that services promote the development of positive emotional and mental health, both as a product of the way they are organised (their process) and through the specific direct initiatives targeted at this goal (their content), using methods such as joint initiatives with voluntary organisations, working with schools, working with health promotion services, developing parent advice services, working with health visitors, working with school nurses and reviewing referral processes
- to ensure that young people, their families and carers are routinely and systematically involved by agencies and are able to express their views on current services and how they would like them to develop, through discussion with users and Tier 1 staff.

The challenges

All Tier 1 professionals have different training, personal interests and anxieties as well as responsibilities. Considerable work will need to be done locally to ensure their ability to think in an inter-agency fashion and have realistic expectations of other professionals and services. All those working with young people should have the ability to develop a strategic plan for any young person and family with whom they are involved.

The fear of being overwhelmed by the demands of other agencies in the locality once a professional is perceived as having special mental health expertise is a challenge to the promotion of Tier 1 work.

Information sharing will raise issues about confidentiality, which will need to be addressed in order that all agencies are aware of each other's involvement with young people. An inter-agency information technology strategy that ensures information sharing will need to be developed, with safeguards.

The locality may be demarcated as the area served by a secondary school with its feeders, or a mental health or social service sector, or the combined catchment area of a group of general practices. School catchment areas seem the most natural localities for children and young people.

Local services will have to be seen as a resource for consultation, training, discussion and support, not just as a referral conduit to the specialist service.

When dealing with the difficult and different predicaments in which children and young people find themselves there are no magic answers. The predicaments require management and all professionals have to own the management strategy. That can be more problematic, especially when the situation is perceived as particularly dire, than passing on the problem to someone regarded as in possession of a magic answer.

There will need to be congruent supervision and management across agencies, so that locality workers are not given conflicting instructions on how to manage their workload in terms of the differing priorities of differing agencies. Line managers must have inter-agency working as their top priority.

Primary mental health workers are seen by some authorities as cheap 'quick fixes' for the ailments of CAMHS. They are not. To function effectively they must have limited catchment areas (maximum 50 000 total populations) if they are to develop useful and trusting relationships and networks. They must be experienced and skilful mental health professionals who command the respect of all Tier 1 professionals in their patch, from general practitioners to headteachers to service managers in social services. They must have good administrative support, so that they can communicate quickly with those with whom they work. They must be closely connected with the local CAMHS, such as by involvement in a Tier 3 team, to avoid isolation and to ensure continuing skill development. The local CAMHS must give absolute priority to referrals from primary mental health workers, as they provide the referral conduit into CAMHS from their locality and they are employed for their judgement on such matters. This will also ensure the Tier 1 professionals with whom they work perceive them as effective. Unless these criteria are fulfilled they will fail and children, families and Tier 1 professionals will be let down.

CHAPTER 12

Liaison and consultation with Tier 1 professionals

Greg Richardson and Ian Partridge

'In the beginning was the word – and the word was anxiety.'
Masserman, *The Practice of Dynamic Psychiatry*

Introduction

The epidemiological evidence is that mental health problems affect 10–20%, and some would say up to 40%, of children and young people in certain settings. If all those children were referred to CAMHS, the services would be overwhelmed. CAMHS see only about 10% of these children. The damage referral can do has been discussed previously, and such a medical way of dealing with these problems is generally not in the children's interests. The alternative of liaison and consultation provides a method of:

* ensuring children with mental health problems, and their families, are dealt with by those with whom they already have a relationship
* reaching more children than could be seen by individual mental health professionals
* increasing confidence and expertise among those dealing directly with young people and their families (Richardson & Partridge, 2000).

Interestingly, neither liaison nor consultation is listed by the Audit Commission (1999) as good practice guidance, which rather clings to a medical model.

The challenges to effective liaison and consultation

The referral system and other perverse incentives

The common factor behind all referrals to CAMHS is the anxiety of the referrer. If this is understood and addressed, it is more likely that confidence will be given to the referrer and hence to the person who is engendering anxiety. Referrals to other agencies or personnel relieve anxiety but also absolve responsibility, and can mean a loss of skills delivered to the child, the loss of a relationship and the stigmatising of the child. Referral may none the less be an appropriate response to the anxiety, but discussion is required beforehand to determine whether this is so.

The ignorance of the involvement of other agencies

The referral system encourages children to be moved within agencies as well as across them, but lack of liaison often leads to an ignorance of such involvement. General practitioners may not be aware that the education support services or social services are involved with a child they refer to health-based CAMHS. The agencies may then be working in ignorance of each other's input, so confusing the family, possibly contradicting each other and multiplying resource use.

Confidentiality

When discussing individual children known to CAMHS, issues of confidentiality arise (Russell, 1996). Local authorities should recognise their obligations concerning confidentiality (Department of Health and Social Security, 1987), although those are more clearly defined when looking at child protection issues rather than issues of educational need (Richardson & Harris-Hendricks, 1996). The advantage of sup-porting Tier 1 professionals through consultation is that it prevents the children from becoming identified patients of the mental health services and hence such confidentiality issues are avoided and the children are not stigmatised.

Resources

An area with a population of 250 000 may have two child and adolescent psychiatrists, two clinical psychologists, a psychotherapist and possibly three community psychiatric nurses. The question arises as to whether eight staff can effectively integrate with ten secondary schools, the feeding primary schools, the pupil support services and the social services department, as well as deal with all other demands from primary care teams. As resources are unlikely to increase dramatically, the development of locality primary mental health worker posts makes such networking not only a possibility but also essential for the effective functioning of the CAMHS.

Poor management of CAMHS

Despite previous recognition, *Children in Mind* (Audit Commission, 1999) revealed poorly integrated and organised CAMHS within England

and Wales. CAMHS remain a small and poorly understood area of the health service, which often fall to the bottom of planning and organisational agendas.

The effectiveness of interventions

Kolvin *et al* (1981) studied four different school interventions with children and young people with mental health problems. There was improvement in all intervention groups, although some interventions were more effective than others. The resource input was large. Interestingly, the consultation interventions, where the pupils had least contact with the outside mental health professional, were the least effective. This is worrying if a consultation and support model is to be promulgated. However, it raises the importance of management strategies being clearly audited and developed in response to evidence of efficacy rather than due to ideology or personal preference on behalf of members of CAMHS or other professionals. It is an important principle of inter-agency work that expectations are both clarified and evaluated. Consultative and liaison interventions with Tier 1 professionals need to be subject to the same critical scrutiny that is given to our clinical interventions.

The stigma of mental health

The general public view is still that the local CAMHS is the place where 'nutters' go, and where families are told it is their fault that their children have difficulties. Mental health remains tainted with 'madness' to pupils, families and teachers. Overcoming such stigma will have to precede effective mental health work and currently ground is being lost among young people (Gelder, 1999).

Principles of consultation

Start where the consultees are

- Clarify the aims of the consultation.
- Clarify the constraints on the consultation.
- Clarify the areas in which the consulters feel their strengths and the strengths of their service lie.
- Clarify the areas in which the consulters feel deficient or bad about their service.

Evaluation

It is important to be able to measure change over time and thereby evaluate the value of the consultation process, for example through the use of a questionnaire and analogue scale developed with the consultees (Richardson & Partridge, 2000).

Process

- Clarify who has the problem.
- Clarify what the young person and family hope to gain from the consultation.
- Identify who else is involved with the child and family.
- Explain that problems are managed, not cured.
- Clarify where the responsibility for change lies.
- Encouragement is more helpful than diagnosis for both patients and consultees.

Relationships, relationships, relationships

Without the development of relationships, the whole exercise becomes a sham; consultation cannot be done by computer.

Liaison with educational staff

In the early 16th century, Sir Thomas Elyot wrote in *The Boke Called the Governor*, 'Lorde God, howe many good and clene wittes of children, be nowe a dayes perisshed by ignorant schole maisters'. Education was stigmatised by Mark Twain in *The Facts Concerning My Recent Resignation*: 'Soap and education are not as sudden as a massacre, but they are more deadly in the long run'. In the past it has been recognised that teachers are second only to parents in affecting children's mental health, for good or ill. However, most teachers are unconscious of their role as mental health workers. For the past 30 years it has been recognised that teachers 'in marking work, assessing personality, streaming, setting and selection ... are determining the whole future of the child, not only his success in school'. As a result, 'The teacher may be subject to impossible demands, being required to ensure success regardless of ability, and having his ability as a teacher criticised on non-educational grounds' (Shipman, 1968).

A major step forward in determining which factors improve a school's effect on young people's mental health was the publication of *Fifteen Thousand Hours* (Rutter *et al*, 1979). Every pupil now leaving school could have benefited from this work, but political and economic dogma and expediency are the uninvited guests that often prevent children from being enriched by research. The fact that schooling affects all areas of children's functioning, including their mental health, seems now to be generally accepted and is helpfully explained in books for the lay public (e.g. Skynner & Cleese, 1994), as well as in publications directed at teachers (such as Young Minds, 1996). The important positive factors required to make a school effective have recently been described (Mortimore, 1995). However, the place of mental health work in school is viewed as cataclysmically damaging by some (Citizens Commission on Human Rights, 1995) and is apparently ignored by others. In developing countries, the effects of pressures to achieve academically on the mental health of pupils is well recognised (Bartlet, 1996).

Obtaining a statement of special educational need from the education authority encourages the process of referral to capture extra resources. However, the Code of Practice on the identification and assessment of special educational needs (Department for Education and Skills, 2001*b*) and the drive to allocate resources according to need without the bureaucratic process of statement preparation go some way to trying to grade input into a child so that both the child and the teacher are supported in meeting the child's educational needs. The involvement of other child care professionals and the clear recognition that child and adolescent mental health advice may be required should encourage integration of services rather than referrals between services.

With the current emphasis on integration, the pressure on teachers to deal with children with special educational needs in large classes is increasing. Techniques for managing children with emotional and behavioural difficulties in the classroom have been described (Howlin, 1994), but there are considerable barriers to implementing them. In an educational system in which academic prowess and the results of Standard Assessment Tasks are the gold standard, teachers, under-standably, are not well motivated or able to put extra effort into the management of difficult and often unrewarding children, especially if the outcomes of such interventions show up in years rather than hours. The result is often the 'Pontius Pilate' quotation: 'We have procedures in school for dealing with misbehaviour, yet X desperately needs the sort of help that we cannot provide.' The more honest (and legitimate) response is: 'X is beyond our understanding and control, and we are desperate to be supported in helping him with his difficulties or we shall exclude him.' Non-stigmatising interventions based on current teacher–pupil and teacher–parent relationships arise from their confidence that they have appropriate and accessible support. When teachers run into difficulties CAMHS should be able to support them so that they are truly able to bridge the 'divide between cognitive and social development' (Dunn, 1996) in the interests of the mental health of pupils.

School nurses are often drawn into these issues in school and appear to gain confidence in their mental health role if they are provided with regular consultation (Richardson & Partridge, 2000).

Liaison with social services departments

Social services may still be referred to as the 'welfare'. Social workers are often objects of both satire and scorn. They are perceived as bearded, sandal-wearing, do-gooders or pathological zealots whose only desire in life is to remove children from the bosom of their caring families. At the same time they allow other children to die brutally in squalor at the hands of the socially deviant, who have been granted understanding at the expense of justice. Nevertheless, the demands upon social services in respect of children are increasing year on year and they have to deal with some of the most damaged and distressed children in our society. Their staffs, particularly in residential establishments, are often under-resourced and under-trained. Management strategies offered to them could be perceived as 'all well and good in theory' but will be ineffective if support in implementing them is not provided.

When the demands made by social services on CAMHS for individual work with these young people are questioned, the CAMHS professionals are perceived as unsupportively avoiding 'problem' children. Social workers, in their search for support, can also be undermined by CAMHS. Their understanding and assessment of a situation are often in danger of being placed in a subordinate relationship to that of the consulting 'expert'. There is a consequent devaluing of professional status and the disempowering and deskilling of that agency on an institutional level. Such a process is also apparent in legal and court work. The generation of such a hierarchy of regard does not facilitate the management of children in their environment and is not an effective and efficient use of resources, although it may bolster the ego and social status of individual CAMHS professionals. CAMHS cannot accept this hierarchy of regard and then complain about referral rates, lack of resources and the inadequacies of other agencies.

Liaison with primary health care services

Primary care services are often disengaged from, if not ignorant of, the many agencies and systems that work with children. Their under-standing of educational support systems is often poor, so they may be manipulated by schools into avoiding using those systems in the hope of getting a more rapid and effective response from a CAMHS. It is helpful to enquire from all primary care referrers where a child is at school and what educational support they are receiving, as well as about the involvement of other agencies. CAMHS contact with those other agencies then enables the support of children and a discussion of the benefits and purpose of a referral to CAMHS.

It is difficult for general practitioners to attend regular consultation sessions; however, primary mental health workers can visit practices regularly to discuss mental health issues and can always ring to discuss a referral they have received. Similarly, telephone discussions with health visitors and general practitioners help develop relationships with CAMHS professionals and increase understanding of mental health issues. All CAMHS professionals have a role in supporting Tier 1 in this regard. CAMHS professionals always must be aware of the difficulties in a surgery of a very emotional, distressed or angry parent or child and be prepared to talk through the management of that situation. General practitioners take continuing medical education very seriously and multi-disciplinary presentations to them reinforce the message that children's mental health problems are rarely managed exclusively by medical methods.

Agenda for the future

National policy

The Department for Education and Skills (2001b) introduced guidance on the identification and assessment of children who have educational difficulties, which often affect their mental health, and on promoting children's mental health (Department for Education and Skills, 2001a). Similarly, the need for child mental health agencies to work closely with the social services departments of local authorities has been highlighted (Department of Health et al, 1999b). The need for inter-agency working and support is now nationally and politically recognised, so that, for example, bids for developments in CAMHS, such as the CAMHS modernisation fund, depend on joint strategies between health services and local authorities.

Appropriate use of resources

Child and adolescent mental health professionals are not primarily educationalists, social workers or primary care managers, and have a limited contribution to make in decisions about usage of appropriate educational tiers, or primary care and social services resources. However, a child who requires Tier 4 educational resources is unlikely not to have mental health problems. Similarly, child and adolescent mental health professionals may have useful contributions to make in the management of a young person with emotional and behavioural difficulties who is being accommodated by a social services department (in either residential or foster care). Again, the integration of services is essential so that child and adolescent mental health professionals working with Tier 1 will know of these children and may be able to contribute to their effective management. Equally importantly, they will develop a relationship with education, health and social services professionals, to facilitate ease of discourse. This will have an important impact upon the deployment of CAMHS resources.

Formalising the forum for liaison

The establishment of regular forums for the Tier 1 agencies has the advantages of recognising both the homogeneity and the heterogeneity of their needs as well as defining clear points of contact and liaison. All disciplines and professionals within a CAMHS may be involved in this work – establishing links with schools, area social work teams, social services residential provision and primary care teams. Such a process has shown some positive results in areas such as professional confidence, understanding of CAMHS functioning, perceptions of support and appropriateness of referral (Richardson & Partridge, 2000).

Use of the primary mental health worker

To overcome children being parcelled as referrals, child and adolescent mental health professionals require close relationships with schools and their support agencies. Primary mental health workers are crucial in this regard. They have a relationship with local schools, possibly through the special educational needs coordinator, health agencies and social services, so they will be aware of all agencies' involvement with young people and will be able to coordinate their involvement by liaison with them. They are also likely to be seen as a source of advice.

Teacher training

The importance of the role of the school and the teacher in the development of the pupil's mental health is not well covered in teacher training. This is an issue that teachers' trainers need to address, as it is an integral part of the teaching process (Department for Education and Skills, 2001a).

The development of protocols for the assessment of child and adolescent mental health problems

Tier 1 professionals often feel at a loss as to how to manage children's mental health problems and all the emotional baggage that goes with them. Giving them a clear strategy for assessing the problem allows them to feel the situation is manageable and expedites discussion of the problem with other professionals. Protocols need developing for each Tier 1 professional group. An example for general practitioners is given in Box 12.1.

Box 12.1 Handy hints for general practitioners

- Try to determine who has the problem (it is rarely the child) and what he or she is really worried about. You can then direct your interventions accordingly.
- What do the family hope to gain from this appointment?
- A telephone call for advice or discussion is often preferable to referral to another service. A primary mental health worker can be very helpful.
- Always ask who else is involved with the child (e.g. social worker, school special needs department, etc.). They may know far more about the child and be in a better position to help than any medical agency. Referring the family back to them may be the most useful intervention.
- Encouragement of what parents are doing right in their child rearing is more effective than diagnosing what is going wrong. Encourage the parents and they will encourage the child; criticise the parents and they will criticise the child.
- Be sure the family want a referral to CAMHS and are not going to be desperately undermined by it because they already lack confidence in their child rearing.
- Schools have support services to deal with educational problems and problems in school. Families should be directed to use them if they are worried about problems in school.
- There are information fact sheets available from the Royal College of Psychiatrists and other sources.

Conclusion

Children's health depends on their physical and mental well-being. Schools, primary health groups and social services have a large part to play in developing that mental well-being, on which children's adult psychological functioning will be based. Child and adolescent mental health professionals have an absolute obligation to assist these professionals in that work, by developing relationships with them. Consultation and liaison provide a regular structure in which these relationships can flourish.

CHAPTER 13

Referral management*

Sophie Roberts and Ian Partridge

'I'm playing all the right notes, but not necessarily in the right order.'
Eric Morecambe

Introduction

Waiting lists in CAMHS are a common cause of distress to children's families, referrers and professionals within the service, and have been shown to increase rates of non-attendance (Subotski & Berelowitz, 1990). To avoid waiting lists and to provide an efficient service, a CAMHS must have an overt prioritisation and allocation process for its referrals. The process of allocation must be based upon managerially realistic and clinically relevant principles. As discussed previously, in the future CAMHS should move away from a system based upon referrals, to one in which tiers are interacting and mutually supporting each other in such a fashion that the notion of referral becomes redundant and working together is integral. The effective functioning of the primary mental health worker will greatly facilitate this process. In the interim, the process of referral and allocation will be the first test of the efficiency of a CAMHS.

Where general practitioners have access to mental health professionals of different disciplines in adult psychiatric services, they tend to refer different patient groups to each professional (O'Neill-Byrne & Browning, 1996). It is uncertain whether these specific referrals are always geared to meeting the patients' needs. Studies have shown that there is a poor level of understanding among general practitioners (Markantonakis & Mathai, 1990; Thompson & Place, 1995; Jones *et al*, 2000; Foreman, 2001) and paediatricians (Oke & Mayer, 1991) of the different roles of disciplines within a CAMHS. General practitioners identify quick access to services as a top priority for them when they refer children and families with mental health issues (Weeramanthri & Keaney, 2000).

---

*This chapter is a revised and updated version of the paper 'Allocation of referrals within a child and adolescent mental health service' published in the *Psychiatric Bulletin* (Roberts & Partridge, 1998)

Allocation meetings

The first structure in managing referrals is an allocation meeting. This should be organised on a weekly basis, at least, to ensure a prompt response to referrers. Allocation should be undertaken by a member of the service who has sufficient seniority and knowledge of the service to command the trust of those to whom the work will be passed. Alternatively there may be a small allocation team of senior members of different disciplines working in the service. Allocation is not a task for a junior member of the administrative team. Whole team séances, where the referral is moved to a member of the service by some sort of mysterious motion, are not appropriate. Neither is a 'bran tub' of a filing cabinet drawer, from which service members take the referrals of their choice, an efficient way of managing young people and their families. The idea that a psychiatrist must initially assess all referrals is anachronistic, devalues the skills of other service members and generates waiting lists.

All referrals, other than emergencies, should be allocated at this meeting. The remainder of this chapter discusses the criteria that will need to be considered.

The service's priorities

The fewer the staff in a CAMHS, the more important it is they have a priority list for referrals. An example is given in Box 13.1. A very small service may say it is going to assess and manage only young people with possible psychotic illnesses and eating disorders and work with young people in, and leaving, care. All other referrals are then returned, as the service is unable to address them. The priority list must be agreed by the CAMHS and made known to referrers.

Box 13.1 Suggested criteria for prioritisation

- Psychotic disorder
- Severe depressive disorder
- Eating disorder
- Obsessive–compulsive disorder
- Emotional or neurotic disorder
- Psychosomatic disorder
- The mental health problems of those involved with social services
- The mental health problems of those involved with education support services.

Urgency

The allocation team, or a member of it, should assess the validity of an urgent referral and allocate accordingly. Referrals of young people who have taken a drug overdose or otherwise seriously harmed themselves should be rapidly processed and seen within 24 hours of being physically fit. Referrals assessed as emergencies should be dealt with immediately by whichever member of the team has time. Certain disciplines (e.g. community psychiatric nurses or junior doctors) should have time for emergencies built into their weekly timetables. Such cases may not reach the allocation meeting but must be recorded as part of the CAMHS workload.

Sector

Sectorisation facilitates close liaison with Tier 1 workers and enables the establishment of networks and relationships with particular members of CAMHS. If referrals are taken only from the primary mental health worker, if one is allocated to that sector, there is an opportunity for effective management of referrals as well as more directly effective liaison with Tier 1 services.

Clarification

Contact between the referrer and the service preceding referral is of considerable help to the allocation team. Indeed, referral may be reframed as a request for consultation. Not infrequently clarification is required and a nominated member of the allocation team should take responsibility for this liaison function and obtain the necessary further information to facilitate appropriate allocation. The involvement of other agencies involved with young people who are referred to the service is often unclear and may require further information from the referrer to avoid duplication of work, or agencies working at cross-purposes.

Inter-agency work

A number of other agencies may be involved with a referred young person and 'ownership' should be clarified. There is the danger, with a number of professionals involved with a young person and family, that confusion can arise as to where responsibility and accountability lie. Consideration and discussion with other involved agencies can minimise such danger. Allocation team members may coordinate the CAMHS involvement, or allocate the task to another member of the service. It may be necessary to organise a professionals' meeting to discuss different agency involvement, current and intended. In such circumstances it is important to ensure efficient use of time and resources, and to clarify and agree boundaries, communication networks and appropriate roles with the professionals from the other agencies. Close liaison with other agencies, both formal and informal, can also lead to more effective use of a CAMHS and increased awareness of its service provision.

Disciplinary function

The nature of the referral may dictate referral to a specific discipline acting as an initial filter. Inter- and intra-disciplinary specialities and areas of expertise and interest should be developed and understood by the allocation team to ensure the individual tailoring of assessment processes and management strategies to meet young people's needs.

Specialist teams

A number of specialist teams may be operating at Tier 3; areas covered by these teams may include eating disorders, bereavement, autistic spectrum disorders, attention deficit disorders, paediatric liaison, risk assessment, and family therapy. Allocation may be direct to such a team or there may be a need for an initial assessment by a professional operating at Tier 2.

Individual workloads

An individual's current workload will be at the forefront of the minds of the allocation team; this promotes team cohesion and enables support for those under pressure of work. Occasionally 'holding operations' or alternative allocations are necessary to protect individuals with too heavy a case-load.

Training requirements

Most CAMHS act as training centres for all disciplines, and training is required in Tier 2 and Tier 3 treatment programmes. Trainees are not service providers and therefore their case-loads should be carefully monitored, but they do require young people and families to be allocated to them to gain their experience and develop their expertise.

Co-working

Many referrals require an element of joint assessment or working that does not fit within the remit of a specialist team. Such ad hoc Tier 3 multi-disciplinary working can enable a fuller assessment as well as provide training, staff support, protection and supervision.

Re-referrals

If a young person is re-referred, consideration should be given to the benefits or otherwise of seeing the same professional again. An alternative Tier 2 professional or Tier 3 team perspective may be indicated.

Awareness of the context of referrals

Contractual obligations to commissioners, general practitioners and primary care organisations, as well as pressure from referrers and families, are recognised as influences upon response rates, and, at times, evaluation and management of such external anxieties will be required.

Conclusion

A process of allocation based upon multi-disciplinary consideration and flexibility allows for the clarification of priorities, and the maximal utilisation of resources, wherein the goals of effective and speedy response and supportive team functioning are facilitated.

CHAPTER 14

Structuring and managing treatment options

Ian Partridge, Geraldine Casswell, Nick Jones,
Greg Richardson and Barry Wright

'Philosophers have merely interpreted the world. The point is to change it.'
Karl Marx, *Thesis on Feuerbach*

Introduction

The routine problems presenting to a specialist CAMHS are likely to be addressed by those working at Tier 2, that is, by an individual specialist mental health professional working with the problem. It would be unfortunate if insufficient emphasis were placed upon the organisation of CAMHS to meet the demands of this everyday work, in the expenditure of energy on the development of high-profile, 'specialist' Tier 3 services. This chapter considers the management of the various treatment options that may be offered by a CAMHS. Treatments, such as group work and family therapy, will often be offered by Tier 3 teams, although service members with relevant skills will do this work as part of their Tier 2 responsibilities. The last section of the chapter considers the specific organisational issues generated by the needs of the sensorily impaired. At all tiers the principles in Box 14.1 will be upheld.

Requisites of a Tier 2 service

'Critical mass' of staff

Meeting the needs of the community and providing a comprehensive range of services requires a critical mass of CAMHS staff with a multi-disciplinary skill mix and a clear recognition of professional function.

Assessment

Assessment represents the first stage of any therapeutic relationship and professionals working at Tier 2 need a clear professional model of assessment in the approach to the referrals with which they deal.

> **Box 14.1** Principles of clinical practice
>
> • Seeing all problems within a developmental context.
> • Seeing all problems within a relational context, avoiding an approach based entirely upon notions of individual pathology.
> • Taking an approach that is focused upon problem solving, and that facilitates and 'fits' with the needs of the young person and family.

Continuum of care

The Tier 2 professional, who will link up with Tier 1 workers, will also be in a position to access and make use of Tier 3 and Tier 4 provision, where required. This highlights the importance of clear networks of communication both within CAMHS and with other agencies.

Training

Staff of all disciplines require access to affordable and relevant training. Training budgets are limited and unequal in their distribution. It may be that units develop alternative funding strategies to support less-well-resourced disciplines. In-house training initiatives and multi-agency and multi-disciplinary training programmes are valuable tools.

Supervision

Professional supervision is a prerequisite for effective professional functioning. Supervision requires consideration of the areas of clinical management and practice, the management of workload and case-load, and personal and professional development. Supervision will usually take place within the hierarchical structures of disciplines in which there are clear lines of responsibility and accountability. Within a CAMHS, cross-disciplinary supervision and support are part of multi-disciplinary working, but cannot replace professional supervision.

Treatment options within a CAMHS

The various treatment options are listed in Box 14.2 and discussed under separate headings below.

Parent support and management

Most families at some stage of their lives need support and advice from others, although this is usually from the extended family and neighbourhood. For those requiring more support than this, a progression

---

Box 14.2 Treatment options

- Parent support and management (including parent training and attachment work).
- Case work and inter-agency liaison.
- Psychopharmacological treatments.
- Behavioural therapy.
- Cognitive therapy (including cognitive–behavioural therapy and motivational enhancement therapy).
- Individual psychotherapy.
- Counselling.
- Creative therapies (including play, music and drama therapy).
- Family therapy.

---

through telephone help-lines, the internet, voluntary organisations and primary care may result in contact with CAMHS. The initial approach is to ask the question 'Whose problem is this – child's, parents', family's or referrer's?' If it becomes evident that the parents do require support, it will be necessary to address three fundamental issues:

- the level of the parents' understanding of the child's developmental pathway.
- the parents' level of awareness of how to manage the child's behaviour.
- the effectiveness of the parents' management, and matters that interfere with that effectiveness.

From this starting point, a template of intervention strategies can be developed, aimed at education, advice on management tactics or even reassurance. If the parents' understanding and awareness of their child's and their own difficulties are being undermined by lack of consistency in their approach to the problem, further questions may need consideration:

- What is the nature of the attachment between parent and child?
- Is there a need for parent training?
- Do the parents fail to manage one or more than one (or all) of their children?
- What models of parenting have the parents experienced?
- Do the parents have a history of loss, trauma or abuse?
- Are there current indications of parental depression or mental health problems?
- Are the parents being adequately mutually supportive?
- Are the parents being adequately supported?

This process enables pragmatism in utilisation of resources and also allows the negotiation of an appropriate package of focused intervention. Consideration needs to be given to the motivation and ability of the parents to undertake a focused piece of work. Before embarking on Tier 2 work, it may be helpful to ask certain pragmatic questions, which are an integral part of user and carer involvement:

- Can the parent manage to attend a clinic or out-patient setting?
- Are there travel considerations that make home visiting a preferred option?
- Are there issues about time off work or school?
- Is there insurmountable stigma attached to CAMHS attendance?
- Are there gender or disciplinary issues in terms of allocation?
- Do the young person and family members consent to the process that is being undertaken?

A careful exploration of the practical issues will often avoid unattended later appointments and will allow the Tier 2 professional to be in a position to match the requirements of the parent, child and family to the most appropriate treatment approach, which could involve any of the following, singly or in combination:

- a behavioural programme
- personal counselling or more general support for the parent
- structural work with the parent (e.g. parent advisor model)
- referral to adult mental health services
- referral to a voluntary agency (e.g. Homestart, New Pin)
- referral to a local authority support programme (e.g. family centre, family aide)
- referral to an appropriate Tier 3 service in relation to parent skills training (e.g. Webster–Stratton Mellow Parenting) or parent–child dynamics (e.g. relationship play group).
- parent training and attachment work.

Guidance is available on which interventions have an evidence base (Fonagy *et al*, 2002; Wolpert *et al*, 2002), but certain conditions and predicaments still present to CAMHS for which there is little evidence of effective interventions. In this situation the above principles (Box 14.1) become even more important.

Case work and inter-agency liaison

Frequently a referral to CAMHS may come from more than one source. These situations commonly arise when a young person's difficulties have created concern and anxiety across agencies. As a result, the agencies respond by referring or otherwise requesting help from CAMHS. In such complex but not uncommon situations mental health specialists often finds themselves key players in managing the case or facilitating inter-agency liaison. While this is not a skill uniquely owned by mental health professionals, they often have considerable experience in providing containment for families and professionals alike in situations involving chronic or persisting difficulties or that incite high levels of anxiety.

Tier 2 professionals can offer containing case work strategies such as:

- the pulling together of all relevant information
- effecting communication between agencies and disciplines
- facilitating professional planning meetings
- providing psychological containment in crises.

Psychopharmacological treatments

While there is an overlap of specialist mental health skills within a CAMHS, multi-disciplinary working requires an acknowledgement of specific therapeutic functions. Certain conditions (e.g. attentional disorders, affective and psychotic disorders) may require treatment with medication. While the psychopharmacological brief will be undertaken by the medical specialist who will retain medical responsibility for the treatment, it is also possible that other Tier 2 workers may be involved in the monitoring of the condition. For example, the use of methylphenidate for attention-deficit hyperactivity disorder may be administered by the general practitioner, with the Tier 2 professional occasionally monitoring the functioning of the child at home and school and offering support and management advice. Similarly, a young person on psychotropic medication may receive relapse prevention work from a Tier 2 professional of any discipline, although often the involved professionals constitute an ad hoc, inter-agency, individually orientated Tier 3 team.

Behavioural therapy

Most Tier 2 workers can be expected to have a working knowledge of behavioural techniques. The role of the therapist is to facilitate a relearning process which examines existing learning patterns, sets new goals and alters behavioural contingencies in order to encourage the building up of desired behaviours. In the absence of more pernicious factors (e.g. abuse, neglect, severe family dysfunction), such techniques are effective and have the advantage of teaching parents the process of managing their child's behaviour rather than just offering a short-term solution to a specific behaviour.

In considering a behavioural approach, the professional should assess:

- the scale of the difficulties – for example whether the behaviours are being maintained by the parental responses and how much motivation to change there is within the family system

- whether the problems are being correctly defined
- whether behavioural treatments are being correctly and consistently applied.

Cognitive therapy

Young people presenting with symptoms caused or maintained by maladaptive cognitive habits or schemata are ideally suited to focused work, which will enable the exploration of the meaning of events and the testing of alternative thinking habits. This approach is of particular benefit for late childhood and adolescence, wherein collaborative work may be used to explore the 'faulty' cognitive assumptions all too common during this developmental phase. It has the value of being focused and short term as well as a problem-solving technique that needs minimal involvement with, and pathologising of, the young person (Graham, 1998). Motivational enhancement therapy may be useful in young persons wishing to address their substance misuse or in those with eating disorders (Schmidt & Treasure, 1993).

Individual psychotherapy

Child psychotherapists are few in number and their work can be time intensive. However, while different psychotherapists may set different referral criteria and work from differing psychotherapeutic paradigms, it is clear that certain groups of young people may benefit from individual psychotherapy, if they have problems such as:

- internalising disorders, such as anxiety
- histories of loss and bereavement
- abusive backgrounds
- struggles with transitional issues
- marked separation difficulties
- difficulties arising from adoption or fostering.

Allied to such work, the ability to offer psychotherapeutic consultation to carers and parents of young people facing difficulties, as well as to fellow professionals operating within and without the service, is recognised as being of value.

Counselling

There is little evidence that individual counselling is effective with children and young people, despite the high demand by parents and adults in the child's world who wish to distance themselves from and pathologise the child. Because of the unequal power relationships between adults and children, such counselling may even be considered abusive.

Creative therapies

Other therapeutic models making additional use of non-verbal mediums such as play, music, art and drama can be helpful options within a CAMHS setting. Alternative methods of working with a child acknowledge the internal and external realities through different media and provide a safe space for a young person to find a way of making sense of and managing traumatic events or inadequate levels of care.

Family therapy

Family therapy can be a labour-intensive treatment option, particularly as it offers an important training function for trainees of all disciplines in a systemic approach to child and adolescent mental health. With limited resources and with increasing demands upon CAMHS, such a provision must be effectively managed and clinically relevant (Partridge *et al*, 1999).

Family therapy should attempt to offer some flexibility as to when it operates and should recognise families' work commitments and schooling. Teams should be of a multi-disciplinary composition, with at

---

Box 14.3 Considerations in allocation to family therapy

- The nature of the presenting problem and its relation to family functioning.
- Family therapy intervention has to be geared to the developmental level of the children, or the children can be excluded if adult issues need addressing.
- The nature and quality of the referral must be considered, especially if reference is made to interactional family factors. Further clarification from the referrer may be necessary to decide the relevance of family therapy.
- The urgency of response required may mean that the family cannot wait for a family therapy appointment. It is, however, recognised that in a crisis family therapy may be effective in helping a family to gain confidence in their own resources rather than their relying on 'help' from outside agencies. Resources would be stretched, however, if emergency family therapy had to be provided.
- Alternative responses may be more effective or economical, such as a visit by a community psychiatric nurse.
- Practical issues for the family, such as access to the service base in terms of transport or financial considerations, need to be examined.
- Any previous contact with the family by the CAMHS may inform the decision as to whether family therapy would be a helpful intervention.
- The recognised indicators and counter-indicators for family therapy should be reviewed (Skynner, 1976; Lask, 1987).

---

least two experienced core members and two regular practitioners, as well as professionals in training. The team should be coordinated by a senior clinician. Referrals will be either direct, from general practitioners, social workers or education personnel through the allocation process, or indirect, via a member of the CAMHS who has already been involved with the family. Families should be asked to confirm their attendance by a given date; similarly, if families fail to attend subsequent appointments a letter requesting their commitment to future sessions may be required. Such a system does increase administrative time, but it enables the service to be more cost-effective. The points to consider when allocating family therapy are listed in Box 14.3.

It may be that, with the development of effective primary mental health worker systems, family therapy teams can be decentralised and developed on an inter-agency basis in localities. CAMHS staff will have a role in this process, supporting the primary mental health worker in the development of the team and in the training of professionals from other agencies.

At times, when it is considered economical in terms of time or useful in engaging a family, a pre-assessment interview or contact by a member of the CAMHS may be used. Consideration of families' expectations and experiences of family therapy is important in the overall organisation of the service to ensure confident engagement by the family. Efforts should be made to keep the families fully informed at all stages of the process, from the information leaflet they receive with their first appointment to decision-making regarding discharge. Monthly appointments for out-patient family therapy are routine in busy services and give time for families to work on issues raised in the session.

Box 14.4 Managing a family therapy service

- Set clear and explicit criteria for allocation.
- All families who appear from the referral to be suitable for family therapy could first be seen by a member of the team for initial assessment and engagement. The 'personal touch' may be more effective than the impersonality of written information to a family in 'need' or 'crisis'.
- Distinguish overtly between seeing a family for family therapy and offering a family assessment.
- Involve the families in the process of treatment, and emphasise clear explanations and engagement throughout treatment.
- Use an opt-in system for appointments, as this reduces waiting times and minimises non-attendance rates.
- Be flexible about activating alternative treatment resources.
- Use a focused, problem-solving model of therapy.
- Establish ongoing evaluation of the service.

Box 14.5 Requirements of sensory impairment service provision

- An established common language across agencies.
- Clear priorities, because resources will be limited. Parents and other service users should be involved in discussions about prioritisation where possible (Green *s*, 2001).
- Realistic goals.
- Avoidance of service duplication.
- Networking with other agencies and teams involved with these children, young people and their families.
- Accessibility.
- Reliable information about the numbers and the needs of children and young people with sensory impairments in the locality served.
- The development of an awareness of, and liaison with, relevant local educational establishments, including special schools (e.g. deaf–blind schools and schools for the deaf).
- The establishment of contact with local communities and community leaders that represent people with sensory impairments.
- Clear delineation of the services that are available and routes of access to them.
- The establishment of ongoing training for specialist teams.
- The establishment of training in the mental health needs of this group of children and young people for other professionals.
- Developing the awareness of commissioners to unmet needs.
- Developing services that are predictable and reliable.
- The coordination of services and links to other local services.
- Staff who are trained in meeting the mental health needs of the sensorily deprived.
- Links to highly specialised services.
- The treatment of families in a culturally sensitive manner.
- Access to a broad range of clinical skills.
- The employment of staff with sensory impairments.

Family therapy has many and varying clinical modalities; a brief, focused and structural model (Minuchin, 1974; de Shazer, 1985, 1988) has many advantages within a busy CAMHS, service delivery being as important as clinical purity. Key points regarding the management of the family therapy service are listed in Box 14.4.

Family therapy is a central service of CAMHS, in that systemic and developmental insights inform all interventions with children and their families. It offers a potent training arena for trainees and new members of staff, and facilitates the development of closer working practices among staff. The opportunity for live supervision also enhances the development of critical and supportive working patterns. Similar organisational principles also apply to the management of a group work service.

> **Box 14.6** Assessment issues in the mental health of children with sensory impairment
>
> - Idiosyncratic, variable or delayed language development (NHS Health Advisory Service, 1998).
> - Stigma (SIGN, 1997).
> - Problems in attachment between child and parent (Stein & Jabaley, 1981).
> - Over-involvement or over-protection (Weddell-Monnig & Lumley, 1980).
> - Polarised or dogmatic approaches to education (SIGN, 1997).
> - Tendency to go on into employment that is below their intellectual ability (Kyle & Pullen, 1995).
> - Difficulties accessing health care professionals (SIGN, 1997).
> - Difficulties communicating with health care professionals (SIGN, 1997).
> - Frustration with communication.
> - Social withdrawal.
> - Aggression and irritation.
> - Selective attention to (or ignoring) the social environment.
> - Learned helplessness.
> - Inadequate seeking of clarification.
> - Generalised 'yes' responses.
> - Delayed social, emotional and cognitive development of deaf children.
> - Poor impulse control.
> - Poor emotional recognition.
> - Under-developed empathy skills.
> - Delayed development of social problem-solving skills (NHS Health Advisory Service, 1998).

Children with sensory impairment

Children with sensory impairment may also have mental health needs and mental illness services should be developed to allow an appropriate response to these needs. For example, there is evidence that the prevalence of psychiatric disorder is higher among deaf children than it is in the general population (Hindley *et al*, 1994; Kyle & Griggs, 1996). Although this may be linked to an increase in organic problems and learning difficulties, it is important that an integrated service approach is developed (Box 14.5). It is important to have a clear definition of which group of children are to be supported by a particular part of the CAMHS. While in principle there should be no need for definitions because children with sensory impairment should have full access to generic services, in practice new services (or a clear rethink about existing services) are the only ways of meeting performance assessment framework targets for this group of children. Children and families should have access to a range of services across the tiered system, depending upon their needs.

It may be that CAMHS establish a Tier 3 or even, due to the specialism of provision, a Tier 4 service to meet the needs of this group. This would have the advantage of giving a clear message that specific needs were being considered and that service delivery was by competently trained professionals experienced in working with this group.

Situating such a service within a generic CAMHS allows for cross-fertilisation of ideas, enables specialist professionals to keep abreast of generic work, avoids the ghetto-isation of the client group and links the child and family into the wider multi-disciplinary service. Assessment (Box 14.6) and treatment need to be evidentially informed, family centred and taking place within the context of clear networking and communicating with other involved agencies.

CHAPTER 15

Paediatric liaison

Christine Williams and Barry Wright

'*What* is the matter with Mary Jane?
She's perfectly well and she hasn't a pain,
And it's lovely rice pudding for dinner again!
What *is* the matter with Mary Jane?'
A. A. Milne

Introduction

Children with mental health problems and psychiatric disorders frequently present in paediatric clinics and wards. Between a quarter and a half of children in paediatric out-patient clinics have conditions in which psychological factors play a major role (Lask, 1994). The arguments for CAMHS input to paediatric services to meet the needs of these children are therefore overwhelming; the benefits are summarised in Box 15.1.

Box 15.1 Advantages of liaison between paediatric services and CAMHS

- A greater understanding of the respective services (Brown & Cooper, 1987; Cottrell & Worrall, 1995).
- Benefits for children and families referred to both services (Schwamm & Maloney, 1997).
- Development of a common understanding and common language relating to the psychosocial aspects of physical illness (Vandvik, 1994), for both career professionals and trainees.
- Greater ability to put family and psychological issues on the agenda (Bingley *et al*, 1980).
- Mental health professionals are kept up to date with paediatric issues (Leslie, 1992).
- The sharing of ideas (Mattson, 1976).
- Opportunities for consultation (Jellenik *et al*, 1981), liaison and the regulation of workload between services (Black *et al*, 1990).

Establishing a liaison team

For a paediatric liaison team to be successful it must have commitment from both paediatric services and CAMHS. A starting discussion between interested representatives from both services should clarify the potential benefits of regular liaison. Both services need to own such a development and discuss its mutual benefits with their staff to ensure their commitment and interest. Liaison meetings without consultant paediatricians have limited usefulness. Exploratory discussions may centre around agenda items such as those listed below:

- Who will meet? Should there be one large meeting for medical and nursing staff, and other specialists such as speech and language therapists, physiotherapists, ward teachers, occupational therapists and liaison health visitors? Alternatively, it may be useful for specific disciplines or teams to have separate meeting times, with, for example, a specific liaison meeting for a paediatric oncology team, paediatric surgical wards (Geist, 1977) or paediatric intensive-care units (Kasper & Nyamathi, 1988).

- When will it be best to meet to ensure that as many of the paediatric team are able to attend as possible? In busy working days it may be hard to find time to meet, hence building on forums that already exist may be the most economical use of time. A useful model may be for the liaison team to join the paediatric team towards the end of their weekly ward round, when the team are already together and issues are fresh in their minds (Black *et al*, 1999).

- What is the purpose of the paediatric liaison meeting and are the staff of both services committed to that purpose? Clarifying the purposes of the team in an operational policy will be helpful.

- How will the meeting be structured to allow maximum benefit for those attending, but ensuring that sufficient time is allocated to discuss complex problems?

- What evaluation or audit processes will be used to assess the functioning of the paediatric liaison service?

- What records will be kept of discussions and agreed actions? Decisions about individual children may be recorded in the children's notes, but the paediatric liaison team may wish to keep a record of consultations. Policy matters will require separate documentation, possibly by continual updating of the operational policy. It will need to be clear who has responsibility for such recording.

Box 15.2 Strategies of liaison

- Establishment of a formal paediatric liaison team within the CAMHS.
- A date, time and place when the paediatric liaison team meets with the paediatric team to consult, liaise, discuss cases and refer between the two services. A separate meeting specifically to discuss psychosocial issues as they affect paediatric out-patients and in-patients may be helpful.
- Transfer of staff (nursing or medical) from one environment to the other on secondment or by mutual arrangement.
- Attendance of CAMHS members at the paediatric grand ward round or educational meetings to discuss patients and topics of mutual interest.
- Telephone or email between teams, either at specified times or on an open-access basis.

The structure of the paediatric liaison team

If there is agreement and commitment to the development of a paediatric liaison team, as with all Tier 3 teams described in this handbook, it should be multi-disciplinary. In practice, the size and make-up of the team will depend on:

- the local catchment population
- the nature of the local paediatric service (e.g. does it have specialist regional responsibility or facilities?)
- the expertise, experience, interests and availability of staff within the CAMHS
- the will of service commissioners to have a paediatric liaison mental health service.

It is recommended that there is a medical member of the team with some understanding of paediatric conditions, as paediatricians will not want to explain the details of each condition from which a child suffers. However, it is important for that medical member to defer to other team members in their areas of expertise, to avoid liaison meetings becoming a doctors' club.

Services are often based on different geographical sites and strategies such as those described in Box 15.2 are required to foster relationships between the two services.

The effects of a paediatric liaison team

More referrals and fewer referrals

Patterns of referral and usage of CAMHS by paediatric professionals change after the establishment of a paediatric liaison team (Black *et al*,

1999). Inter-service discussion provides new ideas and support for those already involved with families and may avert the need for formal CAMHS involvement. It can also ensure that the purposes and benefits of a referral are clarified, by establishing clear objectives for, and questions that may be answered by, the referral. It may also indicate that another agency may be more helpful to the child and family, and so ensure that referrals are directed to the most relevant services. Social services, educational services, health visitors and speech and language therapists may be able to meet the child's needs better than the CAMHS, although a full multi-disciplinary liaison discussion may be necessary to clarify this. A clearer understanding of CAMHS functioning by paediatric professionals, as a result of working with a liaison service, may mean greater use of specialist resources such as the CAMHS Tier 3 teams. Similarly, there may be more referrals for psychosomatic problems (Black *et al*, 1999), reflecting an increased awareness of the psychosocial factors involved with many of these children.

Urgent cases

Good relationships fostered within the meetings help to facilitate the process of urgent referrals in both directions, through understanding and discussion of each other's priorities. Audit of the numbers of urgent referrals can lead to time being allocated prospectively to deal with the work generated.

Joint working

Regular liaison between CAMHS and paediatric professionals permits the integration of psychosocial, psychological and physical interventions, and this helps young people to deal with their illness from a number of different perspectives. This is particularly helpful with children who have a chronic condition such as diabetes, epilepsy or cystic fibrosis, for which joint clinics run by the paediatric staff with a member of the paediatric liaison team may be considered.

Cooperation and mutual respect

Developing relationships in this way provides opportunities for two-way learning, both for professionals in training and for qualified staff (Leslie, 1992). Respect for various working models grows quickly, enriching the quality of service to young people and their families. Where needs are jointly highlighted, ventures such as training workshops, presentations and other multi-agency forums are more easily organised (Williams *et al*, 1999a).

Multi-agency assessment

Joint assessments may be required on an ad hoc basis, whether to clarify a child's needs or as part of a more formal statutory assessment (Sturge, 1989). Joint assessment of specific conditions such as attention-deficit hyperactivity disorder (Voeller, 1991), autism (Ward & Keen, 1998) and psychosomatic illness (Dungar *et al*, 1986) may ensure integrated care packages.

Paediatric liaison in other settings

The opportunities for CAMHS professionals to work with paediatric professionals outside formal paediatric liaison settings include the following:

- multi-disciplinary, multi-agency forums for discussing children with autistic spectrum disorders
- multi-disciplinary work in child protection
- meetings set up to discuss children with complex needs where child health problems (mental or physical) are affecting education or other social functioning, at which representatives from agencies such as school, health and education may be required, in addition to paediatric and CAMHS staff, to discuss, with parental or carer permission, how best to help young people (Williams *et al*, 1999*a*)
- the assessment of children whose needs cross boundaries between child mental health and social services (Wheeler *et al*, 1998)
- on-the-spot teaching from CAMHS members in paediatric clinics (Williams, 1983).

Conclusion

Paediatric services and CAMHS often overlap in their client groups and must work together to ensure that the children they serve have an integrated service in which their mental health needs are understood by their paediatric carers and their physical needs are understood by the CAMHS. Both everyday clinical work and statutory work involve paediatric as well as CAMHS staff. They will work more efficiently to the benefit of their patients if there are formal working arrangements, for which a paediatric liaison service provides a firm foundation.

CHAPTER 16

Day patient services

Rosie Beer

'In summer, when days are long,
Perhaps you'll understand the song.'
Lewis Carroll

Introduction

Early descriptions of child and adolescent mental health day units emphasised five-day 'milieu' provision with a strong emphasis on education and behaviour management (Brown, 1996). Although attempts have been made in the USA and Canada to assess the clinical effectiveness and cost-effectiveness of day attendance (Grizenko & Papineau, 1992; Zimet *et al*, 1994), there is a dearth of such reports in the UK (Creed *et al*, 1997; Goldberg & Collier, 1999). However, a number of recent accounts have begun to explore the planning, organisation and clinical potential of day services that offer a wide range of clearly defined specialised services (e.g. Place *et al*, 1990; Davison, 1996; McFadyen, 1999).

Day patient provision and organisation

Day units can offer assessment and therapeutic services that are more specialised, complex and intensive than out-patient services, while they are still community-based and less disruptive than in-patient admission. Most also have the benefit of educational input. Close liaison with specialised education and social services is central to their work. There is now general acceptance within CAMHS of the central importance of maintaining attachments and working with whole systems if the complex needs of children are to be met. Day units can work with children and young people individually and in groups, as well as with their families and the classroom, while keeping the focus of concern within the community and avoiding the 'out of sight, out of mind' dilemma of in-patient services.

Day services can be diverse, flexible and responsive to local needs, and can provide a wide range of readily accessed programmes for local CAMHS at Tier 3 (see Box 16.1). They may offer part-time attendance

---

Box 16.1 Services offered by day units

- Specialised group work, such as social skills, activities-based, psycho-dynamic, art or drama therapy, communication skills.
- Programmes or groups for particular disorders, such as Asperger's syndrome, anxious school non-attendance, attention-deficit hyperactivity disorder, moderate learning plus social skills difficulties, physical and emotional disabilities.
- Parent groups focused on support and parenting skills.
- Integrated programmes of individual, group, parenting and family work.
- Assessment of complex neurodevelopmental, behavioural and parenting problems.
- Maintenance in the community, or rehabilitation after a period of in-patient care, of young people with psychotic disorders.

---

only, to maximise the range of options available and enable continued school attendance or the involvement of other services. Other day services may be more specialised, providing for rarer or more complex difficulties, and may aim to offer an alternative to in-patient care or special education. Full-time provision (five days per week) or the flexibility to offer this when needed is then usual. Day units can be stand-alone or combined with in-patient services; this often reflects the history of the resource and its influence upon the type of service offered.

There is an organisational and, to some extent, philosophical tension between day and in-patient provision as they operate at Tier 3 and Tier 4. For example, a service organised for part-time attendance and structured individual/group programmes would struggle to meet a need for urgent assessment or more extended contact. Similarly, a service offering full-time attendance for young people with a wide range of complex disorders may have difficulty maintaining group and therapist consistency.

While some day services work with the full CAMHS age range, most specialise in working with either children or adolescents, the cut-off age being usually around 12 years. The target age group will tend to influence the type of service provided – for example, day units for children usually see extensive work with parents (and often siblings) as essential to their work with the referred child. The type of service will also reflect the geographical situation. Day services are limited by distance (i.e. time of travel). Services in rural areas are likely to develop as Tier 3 services, closely linked to the locality CAMHS and providing for their needs, whereas day services in large cities or conurbations may develop more specialised services and draw referrals from a number of neighbouring health districts.

> **Box 16.2** Referral protocol
>
> - Clarity for managers, referrers, day service staff, referred children/young people and parents about the type of service offered and for whom (including clarity about the catchment area).
> - Clear routes of referral and stipulation of who can refer (CAMHS professionals only or also education or social services, or paediatricians?).
> - How, when and by whom decisions are made about whether a referral has been accepted and when a place may be available.
> - Are urgent referrals ever accepted? And if so, what are the criteria?
> - Are management arrangements clear and in line with the local CAMHS?

The model of day service chosen should be clear to potential users (see Box 16.2). The unit's position within the wider CAMHS needs to be embodied in management arrangements for the service as a whole. Day services need to be integrated firmly with the full range of CAMHS so that young people can move smoothly between different parts of the service according to their needs. The role of the unit in relation to other services (especially education and social services) must also be clear, particularly if funding is inter-agency. Points of good practice for day units are listed in Box 16.3.

Staffing

Day services for children and young people with complex needs require an experienced, well-resourced and well-supported multi-disciplinary team if they are to function effectively. Although the composition of teams varies, there is a common emphasis on the need for specialised training, regular skilled supervision and well-maintained inter-agency links. Skills mix is as important as multi-disciplinary balance, and most day unit teams should have members with higher training and qualifications in group work, creative therapies, psychodynamic psychotherapy, play therapy and family therapy, in addition to higher training in child and adolescent mental health. Staffing levels and discipline mixes vary considerably, often as a reflection of the historical development of the particular service; however, ideally staff should include professionals from nursing, occupational and creative therapies, psychotherapy, child and adolescent psychology and psychiatry, plus possibly physiotherapy and speech/language therapy. Teaching staff (funded by the education service) and social work input (funded by social services) are crucial to the type of service offered and to effective inter-agency liaison. Experienced administrative and secretarial support is critical to the smooth running of the service. Stability is aided by

> **Box 16.3** Good practice for day units
>
> - Prompt feedback to a referrer as to whether the referral is suitable for the day service, and if not, possible other sources of help.
> - Minimal waiting times between referral and beginning evaluation, unless referral is for a particular time-limited programme.
> - An initial networking meeting and/or telephone contacts with previously involved professionals to exchange information and clarify the aims of admission to the day service. This meeting may also act as a consultation to the referring professionals, to clarify needs, other possible sources of help and/or other necessary actions (e.g. child protection planning).
> - Initial meetings with the child or young person and family to reach a shared understanding of their needs, the aims of unit admission and expected input from staff and family.
> - Regular reviews while the child or young person is attending the unit and close liaison with school, referrer and other professionals involved. Review meetings may usefully involve family and professionals, so that mis-understandings and 'splitting' can be avoided.
> - Careful discharge planning to ensure continuity of provision by locality CAMHS or other community services.
> - A system for regular feedback on levels of satisfaction with the service from all involved, and constructive evaluation of any complaints or suggestions for change.

some staff working full time in the day service, whereas the presence in the team of members who also work part time in community services will help foster awareness of need and integrated working.

Staffing levels are difficult to stipulate, as working practices and structures vary so widely, but CAMHS day services are specialised and demanding services and not a cheap option. Transport to and from the unit may need to be provided as a routine part of the service, for example for younger children and their parents, for those travelling long distances or where no suitable public transport exists, and for house-bound adolescents for whom attendance independent of their parents is a critical part of their management.

Evaluation

Audit and evaluation can present difficulties, because multiple thera-peutic approaches are often employed simultaneously, family, school and community influences are still active daily, and diagnostic categories may be less clear and less helpful than in other services. In addition, children, young people and parents may deny, distort or exaggerate their difficulties in ways that are integral to the decision to involve day services, but may render many assessment scales invalid. The diversity and patchy availability of day services may make it difficult to relate efficacy to the impact on other services locally and to make meaningful comparisons between units. Nevertheless user, carer and referrer perspectives on the service should be continually assessed.

There have been evaluation studies of day services (Weiner *et al*, 1999), referrer satisfaction surveys (Park *et al*, 1991), attempts to compare the costs and benefits of day services with those of other services (Zimet *et al*, 1994), and discussions of the complex inter-agency aspects of outcome that need to be addressed if the full value of day services is to be assessed (McFadyen, 1999; Weiner *et al*, 1999; Hayter, 2000). As with all services, clarity of aims is a prerequisite of evaluation. Liaison with a wide range of other services is an essential part of the work. A system to record workload must have a way of recognising and valuing time spent in liaison, including on the telephone, emails and so on.

CHAPTER 17

In-patient psychiatric care

Greg Richardson, Geraldine Casswell, Nick Jones
and Ian Partridge

'"It all comes," said Pooh crossly, "of not having front doors big enough".'
A. A. Milne, *Winnie the Pooh*

Introduction

With the development of locality-based and family-orientated intervention in community CAMHS, in-patient psychiatric treatment for
children and young people is rarely required. However, in-patient care is
a specialised field which must continue to be provided if particularly
unfortunate young people with serious psychiatric illness are to be
treated in appropriate settings with skilled and experienced staff.

In England and Wales, the National In-Patient Child and Adolescent
Psychiatric Study (2001) identified 80 child and adolescent psychiatric
in-patient units, providing 900 beds, 73% being managed by the
National Health Service and approximately 12.5% operating on a five-
day week. Bed occupancies range from 40% to 100% and yearly
admissions from 18 to 60; units serve 32 different age ranges, from 0 to
21 with spans of 4–18 years (further details from G.R. on request). The
average length of stay is 74 days, with a standard deviation of 60 days
(National In-Patient Child and Adolescent Psychiatric Study, 2001).
Some units specialise in treating young offenders, eating disorders,
learning disability and neuropsychiatric and psychosomatic disorders,
but most deal with the full range of psychotic, emotional, psychosomatic and eating disorders at the severe end of the range.

Who and what are in-patient units for?

When looking at the criteria for in-patient admission there are a range
of psychiatric, educational, social service, criminal and societal indications. It is usually impossible to separate the different parts so that
each can be provided by the different agencies responsible for it.
Psychological disorders as a result of adverse life experiences are
common and pure psychiatric disorders are rare, but they all have

117

educational and social precursors and sequelae. Indeed, severe psychiatric disorders, such as the pervasive developmental disorders, are managed most usefully by educational interventions. Trying to compartmentalise children into uni-disciplinary treatment pigeonholes is problematic, for the following reasons:

- Residential policies of social services departments tend to address young people's mental health and educational needs only as secondary considerations.
- The Home Office, which will be caring in prisons for a large proportion of young people with conduct disorder and complex needs when they become adults, has little investment in childhood preventive work.
- Education authorities have to meet young people's special educational needs but cannot isolate these from other social and mental health factors, which they do not have the resources to address.
- Admission to psychiatric in-patient units considerably disrupts education and the young person's functioning in the community.

Work on sharing residential responsibility and input requires considerable inter-departmental and inter-agency working, but each agency will be uncertain who is going to reap the most for investing in them, and the harvest is not guaranteed. These issues compound the problems of understanding the purpose of in-patient psychiatric units, because of a lack of clarity about their purpose and function. As a result, in-patient units are bedevilled by:

- the need for proper pre-admission assessments by locality CAMHS to ensure appropriate bed usage
- the difficulties of rapid access, especially in emergencies (Anonymous, 1997)
- a lack of clarity on the criteria for admission
- being seen as the last resort rather than a source of expertise
- the difficulty of maintaining young people's locality links during and after the period of stay, both clinically and managerially
- the need for a respite role for those with psychological developmental disorders such as autism
- the problems over the continuing education of the young people
- a lack of inter-agency agreements on the placement of children for whom they are responsible, when they no longer require in-patient psychiatric care
- uncertainty over whether the in-patient service should provide out-patient follow-up
- lack of information on outcomes and effectiveness
- problems with the recruitment, training and retention of staff

- uncertainty over the transition of young people to adult services or more specialist services.

There is also the need to decide whether an in-patient service should serve a designated area, which would allow the development of relationships with locality CAMHS in that area and hence tailored in-patient interventions, or whether the in-patient unit should serve a far wider catchment area and provide treatment for specific disorders, such as psychosis or eating disorders. The latter would allow the development of very specialist expertise but at the cost of relationships with locality CAMHS, as too many of them would be relating to such a specialist service.

Integrating in-patient treatment into a continuum of care

Only by considering admission in terms of the young people's developmental needs and their progression through a continuum of management will the demand-led adolescent in-patient services of the USA (Bickman et al, 1996) be avoided. In the UK, community working has replaced much in-patient care and this trend is echoed in the decline of residential child care and residential education. It is now increasingly recognised that a period of in-patient care is just one part of the care pathway, which must always be preceded by the comprehensive assessment of young people as soon as they come into contact with the CAMHS. During admission, close communication and joint working are required between the in-patient service and the locality service. This ensures continuity of care of the young person before, during and after an in-patient stay and should secure comprehensive, planned community provision on discharge. Discharge planning should occur well before a young person is admitted to an in-patient unit so that the in-patient care becomes a part of the total care package and not an isolated, short-term, problem-solving, disruptive event in the young person's life. This requires agencies to take responsibility for smoothing the care pathway so that the in-patient work with the young person is undertaken in the context of family and local professional networks.

Admission criteria

Although experts in the USA have reached a reasonable degree of agreement on which adolescents require residential care (Strauss et al, 1995), namely those with conduct disorder and a history of substance misuse, few British psychiatrists consider that such young people would benefit from psychiatric admission. In the UK, the criteria for admission to children's units are changing fairly quickly (Bhui & Moran, 1995) and the work of such units has been well described (Green & Jacobs, 1998).

Adolescents, although rarely children, occasionally suffer serious psychiatric illness, which requires their care in a safe, monitored environment. Care on wards with adults who are psychiatrically ill is widely recognised as harmful. There is therefore a need for a ward for psychiatrically ill adolescents, which has as its indications for admission:

- psychotic disorders
- major depressive disorders
- eating disorders unresponsive to other treatment
- emotional disorders that are incapacitating
- psychosomatic disorders that threaten life or development.

If resource availables are there may be a place for the Department of Health to run therapeutic communities, but this must take second place to providing for the psychiatrically ill.

Adequacy of in-patient provision

The data from the National In-Patient Child and Adolescent Psychiatric Study (2001) showed that bed provision in England and Wales varied from 1.7 to 6.5 beds per 100 000 people aged under 18 years, but there was no indication regarding what the optimum level may be. London, where there is considerable difficulty accessing beds, is at the top end of the range, with 5.5 beds per 100 000. Needs assessment would indicate that there are likely to be higher incidences of serious psychiatric disorder in deprived inner-city areas, but still the bed requirements are so small that estimates are difficult. Initiatives in other areas, such as the Early Intervention in Psychosis processes promulgated in the National Service Frameworks for Working Age Adults with Mental Illness, may have a significant impact on the needs for beds for adolescents.

Effectiveness of in-patient provision

The data from the National In-Patient Child and Adolescent Psychiatric Study (2001) included the average length of stay, which may be used as a comparator, but there is no evidence that this reflects an optimal length of stay. Audits across different in-patient facilities of different patient groups should contribute to available data. In the meantime, robust admission and discharge policies should ensure as effective use as possible, within the limits of current knowledge.

Alternatives to in-patient care for young people suffering from a serious mental illness

Efficient use of in-patient resources depends on comprehensive community CAMHS. Community CAMHS may develop intensive-care teams to enable them to look after seriously ill young people in their homes. This is an expensive option but prevents the extra disruption to the young person's life of removal from home. Certain disorders, such as anorexia nervosa, may be cared for on paediatric wards, if the local paediatric team is prepared to take this on, and if they are fully supported by the locality CAMHS. This may prevent a young person having to be admitted a long way from home.

Increasing awareness of an in-patient service

Because in-patient units have large catchment areas, it is difficult to maintain constantly communicating relationships with all potential referrers. Overt admission, discharge and operational policies must be widely disseminated and updated in the light of experience from referrers, users and their carers, so all know what they can expect from the service.

Organisational issues

Each Tier 4 service should have a designated catchment area commensurate with its bed capacity. Each unit should then be able to respond to all requests for admissions in the following circumstances:

- The young person is suffering from an acute psychiatric disorder.
- The young person has been assessed by a consultant in child and adolescent psychiatry, who is requesting the referral. This should ensure that the young person has been fully assessed as requiring psychiatric in-patient assessment, treatment or management and that such assessment, treatment or management is not possible in the community.
- The young person meets the overt admission criteria of the in-patient unit.
- The unit has a contractual commitment to the relevant commissioning authority or primary care organisation, the commissioning authority having agreed how many in-patient psychiatric beds it requires for the young people for whom it is responsible. Such contracts are the only way the provision of in-patient services can be guaranteed.
- The place to where the young person will be discharged is clear.

Discharge planning is an integral part of in-patient care and is the vehicle that ensures the period of in-patient care is as short as possible and is part of an integrated package of care. Community CAMHS as well as local education and social services must therefore give high priority to discharge planning meetings and Section 117 meetings held by the Tier 4 facilities. The Care Programme Approach (CPA) (Department of Health, 1990) provides a useful model for this, which should be used with all young people hospitalised in a psychiatric ward.

- The local CAMHS has made a commitment to attend reviews and discharge planning meetings held on the young person at the Tier 4 centre.

In-patient services must ensure that lengths of stay are the minimum possible, by implementing the above and:

- restricting therapeutic input to problems defined at admission
- clarifying the aims of admission, which cannot be achieved in a community setting.

The in-patient unit must be managed by an adequately staffed, multi-disciplinary team (Royal College of Psychiatrists, 1999b) who regularly review progress and provide multi-professional insights and interventions. Each team member must have clear lines of accountability, responsibility and supervision. The effectiveness of any in-patient unit is largely dependent upon the work of the in-patient nursing team, both qualified and unqualified. They provide the day-to-day care, create the therapeutic milieu and provide all the background information that contributes to the 24-hour assessment and treatment of the young people. The majority of nursing staff should have undertaken recognised training in child and adolescent mental health, such as the ENB 603 course. Individual training programmes for each team member should be instigated through annual review. The multi-disciplinary team must meet regularly (probably weekly as a minimum) to discuss the progress of in-patients, and at a separate meeting discuss policy and operational issues; there is also a need for systemic discussion about the functioning of the service.

A key worker or primary nurse system should be in place, to ensure that there is one member of staff who takes responsibility for the planning of the day-to-day care of the young person and to ensure that this is integrated with the treatment plan. The key worker is then the focus for communication by the young person, the family, the involved community professionals and the other members of the in-patient team. The young person and family should always be informed who is standing in as key worker when the key worker is off duty.

In-patient services should provide written documentation to the referring community CAMHS on the findings and agreements arising from the pre-admission assessment, a report on the initial assessment review, after the initial period of in-patient care, regular (e.g. six-weekly) reports, the notes of all discharge planning meetings and a discharge summary.

Each in-patient service should have developed evidence-based protocols for the management of conditions that cause young people to be admitted to that service.

The in-patient unit must have a comprehensive operational policy. This should allow the preservation of a bed in each unit for emergency admissions. However, psychiatric emergencies in young people are rare, so such young people should be thoroughly assessed locally by child mental health professionals as suffering from a psychiatric disorder before a referral is made. The only real psychiatric emergency is an acute-onset psychosis. Young people cachectic from an eating disorder may best be cared for on a paediatric or medical ward, in order to ensure their metabolic stability, before being transferred to an in-patient facility, which should be achievable with some rapidity. The period while the young person is on the medical ward gives the family time to become acquainted with an in-patient facility and its staff and to decide whether they consider transfer is going to be helpful. Deliberate self-harm provides a high-risk situation, but comprehensive community assessment and management should precede admission and the young person and family or carers should be given ample opportunity to visit, talk about and discover the pros and cons of in-patient admission. Keeping a bed for emergencies should not interfere with a desirable bed occupancy rate of 80–85%.

Substance misuse is increasingly common among young people and cannot be used as a reason for the exclusion of a young person from an in-patient service if the psychiatric state justifies admission.

An adolescent psychiatric in-patient facility must operate for seven days a week, 52 weeks a year, as the severity of disorder and level of dependence of these young people, when they are acutely ill, is such that it is not safe to place them elsewhere at weekends.

Such a facility must be able to cope with young people detained under the Mental Health Act. Staff must therefore be trained and have up-to-date knowledge of the Act.

Children under 11 years very rarely require psychiatric admission, and such admission should not be used to deal with extreme aggressive behaviour, bearing in mind that children are further damaged by prolonged distant removal from their homes and communities. Those under eight years should probably not be admitted without their family in view of the importance of attachments at younger ages.

The optimisation of local facilities, to avoid in-patient psychiatric care, must be considered. For example, young people with eating disorders may be looked after on a paediatric ward with intensive support from a CAMHS. A Tier 3 eating disorders team that involves paediatric as well as CAMHS staff may be effective in reducing the need for in-patient psychiatric provision for these young people if in-patient provision is provided on the paediatric ward. Similar CAMHS support may also help in the management of young people with complex psychosomatic problems on paediatric wards.

The problem of professional isolation in in-patient units has to be addressed by ensuring that these professionals also work in community CAMHS or that the different tiers occupy adjacent premises so there is regular contact between staff working at the different tiers.

In-patient units of fewer than 10 or 12 beds become very expensive per bed because it is not possible to have proportionately fewer staff. For example, there will always need to be at least two staff on at night and three throughout the day, whether there are four or ten young people on the unit.

Whatever the local provision, there may still need to be an occasional very specialist placement for forensic or neuropsychiatric purposes or when local services have not been able to manage the young person's illness successfully.

In-patient services should not disempower locality CAMHS by automatically offering follow-up care of in-patients and taking over the community and out-patient care of patients referred to them, unless this is clearly negotiated with the referring service. Equally, community CAMHS must recognise that in-patient care is part of a pathway of care which begins and ends with them.

Consideration may be given to the appointment of Tier 4 link workers to community CAMHS. Their job would be to develop close relationships with Tier 4 staff and to help young people and their families in the transition to and from Tier 4 facilities. They might also be involved in therapeutic interventions with the young people for whom they are responsible, at the Tier 4 site.

Support and assistance for the families of young people resident in in-patient facilities, especially with regard to transport, should be considered.

An agreed protocol should be developed for the transfer of care of young people from adolescent in-patient services to adult mental health services when required.

All in-patient services should have robust clinical governance processes. These will include risk assessment being undertaken for each young person admitted, a process for investigating serious untoward incidents and regular sessions (e.g. half a day every two months) for multi-disciplinary audit. The consent, or lack of it, of young people and their carers must also be recorded and regularly reviewed. Clinicians working in different in-patient facilities should be encouraged to meet to develop common priorities, service standards and outcome measures, and audit them.

An agenda for the future

Standardisation of the age ranges accepted by general in-patient units is required in order that referrers and commissioners can have a clearer understanding of the function and capacity of their local units. Only specialist units should vary from such age bands.

Similarly, the admission criteria for general in-patient units need to be standardised so they can be understood by health professionals and by other agencies. Only then will unrealistic expectations be recognised and appropriate young people be referred for effective treatment.

In-patient units should develop strategies to meet the standards now being recognised nationally (Quality Network for In-patient CAMHS, 2001; Royal College of Psychiatrists' Research Unit, 2001).

There should be permanent, finance-backed agreements that ensure guaranteed beds (when required) to those who have made a financial commitment to the existence of the in-patient unit. Such agreements should also ensure that commissioners can influence service provision and standards. With such an agreement, the referring community service can develop relationships with the in-patient team over time, so improving transition for patients and families between community and in-patient care. From the providers' point of view, the viability of the unit is assured and they develop links with the community staff with whom they have an agreement.

Bed occupancies of less than 80% are not acceptable if in-patient units are to work efficiently.

Psychiatric illness meeting the criteria for admission detailed above is rare in pre-pubertal children. None the less, for such patients there may need to be a facility for family admissions. There are probably more contraindications than indications for the psychiatric admission of the under age of eight without a parent.

Specialist training of nurses in child and adolescent mental health is required to ensure that young people on in-patient units are cared for by staff who understand their illness in the context of their development and environment.

CHAPTER 18

Deliberate self-harm

Barry Wright and Greg Richardson

'It isn't as if there was anything wonderful about my little corner. Of course for people who like cold, wet, ugly bits it is something rather special, but otherwise it's just a corner'
A.A. Milne, *The House at Pooh Corner*

Introduction

Approximately 7% of adolescents harm themselves at some point and 20% will think seriously about it (Andrews & Lewinsohn, 1992). This represents a considerable workload for CAMHS, both numerically and in terms of the risk they pose and the levels of anxiety they generate, although many such young people do not reach the attention of health services (Garrison, 1989). It is the responsibility of CAMHS to assess and manage these young people, as well as the anxiety they engender in others. Around 0.5–1% of young people complete suicide, and 40% of those who survive a first attempt will repeat it. CAMHS should aim to reduce these figures, if at all possible. Suicide has long been recognised as a societal phenomenon as well as an individual one (Bakwin, 1957; Durkheim, 1970) and national strategies are being developed to address this (Department of Health, 2002*a*).

Such young people may be referred to a CAMHS at a number of points in the cycle of self-harm (Box 18.1).

Box 18.1 Referral routes

- From a general practitioner or other professional who is concerned about the possibility of self-harm because of stated intent or a history of self-harm, although less than a tenth of self-harm referrals to CAMHS come in this way (Nadkarni *et al*, 2000).
- From the accident and emergency department soon after an episode of self-harm.
- From a hospital ward after admission for deliberate self-harm.
- After discharge from hospital following an episode of self-harm.
- For in-patient care because of recurrent self-harm, serious suicidal intent or a life-threatening suicidal attempt.

Providing a service

The assessment of the young person is part of the everyday work of CAMHS. It generally requires a speedy response to alleviate anxieties. Alacrity is more important than the professional background of the assessor. Commonly it is a psychiatrist who undertakes the assessment. This is odd, since junior psychiatrists on a rota often have the least experience of child and adolescent mental health problems of all CAMHS members. Some services have one or two members who do all the assessments and who consequently acquire considerable skills. Other services use all members or have a specifically designated Tier 3 self-harm team. Which of these occurs in any particular area is largely dependent on:

- the size of the CAMHS
- the perceived and actual roles and expertise of different members of the service
- the personalities, interests and anxiety levels within the service
- the workload, working patterns and training requirements of different disciplines
- availability of supervision
- the way in which the term 'multi-disciplinary' is interpreted within the service.

In work with adults who harm themselves, research shows that, with appropriate training, many disciplines can undertake the assessments, provided supervision and inter-disciplinary support are available. Clinical and epidemiological information is readily available to inform practice in the management of deliberate self-harm (Rutter, 1985, 1987, 1990; Kerfoot, 1988; Andrews & Lewinsohn, 1992; Harrington, 1994; Kerfoot *et al*, 1996; Geddes, 1999).

Assessment and management

CAMHS, accident and emergency departments and paediatric services should have a clear, mutually agreed protocol for managing these young people (Box 18.2), one that ensures a clear and rapid care pathway. The aim should be that all young people who harm themselves are properly assessed and managed.

Young people (under 16 years of age) should be admitted to hospital when they have made a deliberate attempt to harm themselves (Royal College of Psychiatrists, 1982). This allows for:

- adequate assessment of mental state, both by ward staff observing over a period of time and by a visiting member of CAMHS

Box 18.2 Managing those who self-harm

- Full psychosocial assessment.
- Formulation of recent events (acute, chronic, behavioural disturbance).
- Mental state examination.
- Comprehensive risk assessment.
- Strategies for prevention of recurrence.
- Intervention and follow-up.
- Liaison with families and relevant agencies.
- Preparation and provision of reports.

- time to obtain further information, from family, school, general practitioner and social services (Garrison *et al*, 1991). About a third of young people who harm themselves and present in accident and emergency departments are not accompanied by close family, and a fifth present on their own (Nadkarni *et al*, 2000)
- a cooling-off period for the young person and family, particularly where family breakdown has occurred (this may produce the opportunity for discussion of the reasons for the episode; conversely, it may allow time for the reasons to be repressed and not disclosed, potentially leading to a further episode of self-harm)
- observation of medical condition, particularly with respect to those who may have lied about the severity or nature of self-harm;
- time for professionals to engage with the young person and family or carers to smooth the path for any further care;
- time to set up an adequate intervention package (e.g. medical treatment, family meeting, psychosocial follow-up, social services involvement, school involvement).

Strategies for the prevention of recurrence: intervention and follow-up

Young people who harm themselves are notorious for not attending follow-up appointments and this makes it difficult to evaluate the effectiveness of interventions. However, there is evidence for the efficacy of certain structured interventions, albeit which are primarily, but not entirely, based on research with adults. These include:

- treatment of psychopathology, including the alteration of maladaptive cognitions (Linehan *et al*, 1991)
- improving social skills, problem-solving skills and care-seeking behaviours (Schotte & Clum, 1987; Lerner & Clum, 1990; Salkovskis *et al*, 1990; McLeavey *et al*, 1994)
- facilitating adaptive affect regulation (Lewinsohn & Clarke, 1990)

> **Box 18.3** Enhancing service provision
>
> - Development of a Tier 3 deliberate self-harm team, which can take responsibility for assessment and the delivery of comprehensive management packages.
> - Consultation with other professionals concerned in the care of children who may harm themselves.
> - Advice on the prevention of suicide or further self-harm.
> - Input into the planning of services for those who self-harm.
> - Planning organisational change to maximise effectiveness.
> - Auditing the care and experience of young people who harm themselves.

- family interventions (Kerfoot *et al*, 1995; Harrington *et al*, 1998)
- contracting for no suicidal behaviours, which appears to depend for its success on the patient being able to contact a mental health professional (Rotherham, 1987; Morgan *et al*, 1993)
- brief, structured treatment in the home, which is cost-effective as routine care (Byford *et al*, 1999)
- networking and advice to other agencies that plan or run crisis hotlines (Evans *et al*, 1999), educational programmes (e.g. school or media based)
- opportunity restriction strategies.

Suggestions for enhancing service provision more generally are given in Box 18.3.

CAMHS are sometimes asked to become involved when parents or carers have harmed themselves, and this requires CAMHS to work closely with colleagues in adult mental health services and social services. Similarly, the consequences of parental suicide may require CAMHS involvement (Wright & Partridge, 1999).

Recording

Episodes of self-harm should all be recorded by all involved departments, partly in order to monitor practice. Such data may be collected in the accident and emergency department or by a paediatric liaison health visitor. Paediatric wards and night admission wards attached to accident and emergency departments should also keep figures of admissions for self-harm. These figures should correlate with the referrals to CAMHS as a result of self-harming behaviour. A regular audit should be conducted into the flow of young people through the system to ensure they all receive a service, as, historically, not all children who harm themselves are referred to a CAMHS for assessment (Davies & Ames, 1998; Hurry & Storey, 2000).

Teaching and training on the management of self-harm

Members of CAMHS assessing young people who have harmed themselves will require initial training to recognise the factors associated with self-harm (Kerfoot *et al*, 1996) and in risk assessment. They will subsequently need supervision to discuss their findings and management plans. CAMHS members may be part of paediatric liaison teams and this will allow for discussion of young people who have harmed themselves with colleagues working in general hospital settings, which will also extend the psychological training of those working in such settings.

CHAPTER 19

Learning disabilities services

Christine Williams and Barry Wright

'For the world's more full of weeping than we can understand.'
W. B. Yeats

Introduction

Approximately 1% of the general population has some form of learning disability (Hatton, 1998). The prevalence of severe learning disability (IQ < 50) is 3–4 per 1000, and that of moderate learning disability (IQ 50–70) is 30–40 per 1000 (Felce *et al*, 1994).

Children with learning disabilities are at increased risk of developing mental health problems. The incidence rates quoted in various studies are between 40% and 77% (Corbett, 1985; Wallace *et al*, 1995; Gillberg *et al*, 1986). Children with learning disabilities are also at increased risk of having specific disorders such as autistic spectrum disorders (ASD) and hyperkinetic disorder (Rutter *et al*, 1970). Behaviour that presents significant challenges is estimated to occur in 8–14% of children with these difficulties (Kiernan & Kiernan, 1994).

Services for children and young people with learning disability and their families have often been patchy and inadequate. Recently, a number of documents have been published that recognise the paucity of services for this group (Mental Health Foundation, 1997; NHS Executive, 1998; Department of Health, 2001c). The Royal College of Psychiatrists' report (1992b) recognised the lack of speciality provision for children with learning disabilities and recommended the development of services that include the assessment and diagnosis of complex cases, the prevention and amelioration of mental health problems, specialist treatment interventions and multi-agency liaison.

The Nuffield Institute's Community Care Division (Abbot *et al*, 1998) argues that, due to limited research about this population, knowledge is 'patchy' and what is known is not often shared between agencies. In particular, they say that little is known about children with disabilities who may need to access services as a result of emotional, behavioural or mental health problems. The paucity of literature in this area renders it difficult to know which services routinely treat children with learning disabilities for emotional and behavioural problems.

Box 19.1 Service principles

- Children with disabilities 'should be provided for as children first and people with a disability second' (McKay & Hall, 1994).
- Services for children with learning disability must fit into an organised and structured framework.
- Service delivery must be sufficiently flexible to ensure multi-agency working, liaison and consultation.
- Links with other agencies providing services for these children and their families must be maintained.

Valuing People (Department of Health, 2001c) recognises the need for early identification of impairments and early interventions, coordinated services, family support and continuity of care in the transition to adult services.

The organisation of services

It is first necessary to decide whether mental health services for children and young people with a learning disability will be part of children's services or of learning disability services. Historically, this has varied. Some argue that learning disability should not exclude children from access to the facilities available to children and families in general. Alternatively, some provision is within 'life span' services for people with learning disabilities across all age ranges. Continuity of care is then ensured between childhood and adulthood. In making these decisions, each locality must address the service principles outlined in Box 19.1.

Service considerations

In developing a service based on the principles set out in Box 19.1, consideration will have to be given to the following:

- *The historical situation.* Has the service been traditionally provided in one setting (e.g. a life span service) or does the retirement of a leading professional, such as a consultant, mean that the situation can be reviewed?
- *The allocation of resources.* Is one service rather than another funded to deliver the service and is it feasible to move those resources? Children with learning disability who have no resources to meet their mental health needs require their plight to be made known to those responsible for commissioning health services for them.

- *The management structure of the provider.* It is possible that services for these children may be provided from different departments or directorates within one trust or from different trusts. The relationships and working practices of the different departments and trusts will have a considerable bearing on how the service is delivered.
- Staff expertise may be based in one department and not in another. Negotiations may then be necessary if staff are to move to another department.
- Staff working in different areas have different working practices and those practices may have to be addressed if new ways of working in different organisational settings are to be achieved.
- If existing service configurations are to be changed, the arguments for the change must be clear, with tangible benefits for children and their families.
- National guidance and local strategic thinking may well indicate the most useful management organisation.
- As with all CAMHS, accessibility to services for all those requiring them must be a paramount consideration.

In the light of these considerations, each locality will have to look at the specific advantages and disadvantages of placing the service within CAMHS or learning disability services (Box 19.2).

Work with children with disabilities involves long-term interventions and inter-agency work with large numbers of other professionals. The children frequently have complex needs; interventions with them can be intricate and time consuming, and families may be difficult to discharge (Green *et al*, 2001). Many parents require time and support in coming to terms with the losses associated with having a child with a permanent disability. Some parents, including those who have learning disabilities themselves, need advice throughout the child's developmental stages. In addition, intervention programmes take time to produce relatively small changes.

In order to cope with the huge demands placed on services, strategies for managing workload will have to be considered. These may include:

- keeping to problem-focused, goal-directed work as far as possible
- seeking to utilise empowering interventions that avoid service dependency and that help families to develop the skills to deal effectively with future difficulties as they arise
- targeting and rationing any long-term work to high-risk families
- establishing sharing of work between agencies, particularly with high-risk families.

In this way, parents and staff are encouraged to develop skills and strategies that can be generalised to new problems.

Box 19.2 The placement of a service for children with a learning disability and a mental health problem

Advantages of being within learning disability services

- Staff are trained and experienced in dealing with people with learning disabilities across all ages and are familiar with the disorders from which they suffer.
- There is continuity of care for young people as they become adults and they do not have to cope with a change of service and support personnel.
- Staff are familiar with the agencies, statutory and voluntary, that deal with people with learning disabilities and can access them on behalf of their patients.

Disadvantages of being within learning disability services

- Training staff to treat people across a broad age range – through understanding their developing needs and the different requirements of the different ages – is very demanding.
- Maintaining links with child agencies such as CAMHS and child development centres cannot be a priority when links with adult agencies must also be maintained.

Advantages of being within CAMHS

- The clientele have access to full tiered service provision.
- Links with other agencies, such as social services, education, child development centres and voluntary agencies, working primarily with children, are already established.
- Premises are centred on services for children and young people.
- Children are seen as children first rather than as individuals with disabilities.

Disadvantages of being within CAMHS

- It may be difficult to find trained staff where, historically, service provision (and therefore training) has been part of a separate 'life span' service.

There is an argument that children who have specific diagnostic requirements, complex needs and who may require expert interventions may benefit from seeing members of the team who have experience in the area. It is unlikely that all members of a CAMHS would be in a position to develop this expertise. Much of this thinking leads to the conclusion that certain members of the team may be better placed to take such referrals. They may then form themselves into a Tier 3 team, a 'CAMHS learning disability team', that has a specific role in developing relationships with other clinicians seeing these children, developing liaison and keeping themselves up to date on clinical practice in the area. This gives a focus for consultation, liaison, referral and multi-agency working. However, not all the children with a learning disability who are referred to CAMHS need be taken by the Tier 3 team. There would be flexibility in how wider team members may rotate in and out of the team, in either the short or longer term, to meet the needs of particular children and their families.

A Tier 3 learning disabilities team can help to create a specialist facility within a system, which is able to provide access to a wide variety of other services, to the benefit of families. It does this by integrating the service into a CAMHS and avoids stigmatisation or isolation from other services.

In addition, differentiated funding and commitment to services can protect a service that historically has had a tendency to be eroded by competing needs within host organisations.

Establishing a new service

Where a new service is being created, the generation of a new team creates exciting opportunities for the development of inter-agency relationships. It is an ideal time to bring together representatives from parents' groups and all of the professionals with whom the team would like to establish links, in order to brainstorm with them potential options for the configuration of the service (Green *et al*, 2001). Once a list of potential services have been generated, the group can be asked to reach a decision about the level of priority they feel should be given to each element of the service.

The process as well as the product of such meetings can be valuable in laying the foundation of a service aimed at creating strong links with parents and professionals. It also creates a joint understanding of the demands and limitations of the service.

Once a service has been developed, it will need to address the issues raised in Box 19.3.

Box 19.3 Service considerations

- How new services will relate to existing services?
- How will the new service work in practice and develop its operational policy?
- How will training needs be met?
- Who will be the users?
- How will discrimination be avoided?
- How will the service be audited and monitored?
- How will users' and carers' views incorporated into its practice?

Team structure

The team composition should reflect the multiple needs of children with learning disabilities (Joint College Working Party, 1989; Mental Health Foundation, 1997; Department of Health, 2001c). Most CAMHS do not have the luxury of a large multi-disciplinary team, and some harsh decisions need to be made when constructing a team. There will be a tension between a need to have a range of services and a need to get through the large volume of work. The team will need to consider the range of treatments available, as well as team morale and evidence-based comparison of the effectiveness of the various treatment approaches, efficiency and user/carer experiences. There should also be strong links with professionals who are not part of the core team, including:

- community paediatricians
- paediatricians with an interest in neurology
- school doctors
- school nurses
- social workers and family workers within social services health and disability directorates
- voluntary agencies
- respite care facilities
- educational psychologists and behaviour support services within education
- health visitors.

Referral process

Referrals can be taken from a number of sources, including general practitioners, hospital doctors, school doctors, health visitors, educational psychologists, behavioural support teachers and social workers, who all should be clear about the purpose and functioning of the team. This may require considerable educational input. Criteria for allocation to the learning disabilities team of referrals into CAMHS should be clear from the operational policy of the team. Different services have used differing criteria with varying degrees of flexibility, as outlined in Box 19.4.

A large proportion of children with ASD do not have low IQs or attend special schools. However, professionals working with children with learning disabilities often work with less able autistic children and have developed skills in assessment and management that are valuable throughout the full range of ASD. Hence it may be useful to include ASD within the referral criteria. However, increasing awareness and understanding of ASD have recently led to marked increases in

Box 19.4 Referral criteria

- Attendance at a special school.
- Autistic spectrum disorder.
- IQ below 70 or severe developmental delay.
- Statement under the Education Act 1981 of special educational need relating to learning disability.
- Developmental delay as judged by paediatric/child development centre teams.

referral rates and this must be given careful consideration in the planning of service provision.

Approximately 2% of children have statements of special educational need, although not all of these relate to learning disability. However, the team will have to make calculations to determine the number of children statemented because of their learning disability and how their needs will fit with available resources. Furthermore, liaison should be with all primary and secondary schools rather than being limited to special schools, and this will have resource implications.

This is particularly pertinent because many local education authorities have implemented inclusion policies. In practice, the first two criteria listed in Box 19.4 create a great deal of work, and are more likely to identify children with complex needs, where a specialist service can be most usefully targeted.

Role of the learning disabilities team

A CAMHS learning disabilities team might be expected to perform the following functions:

- assessment and treatment of child mental health problems in children with learning disabilities
- involvement in the assessment and treatment of the mental health problems and disorders of children attending the child development centre, through close links with paediatric and child health teams and the provision of consultation to them
- offering behaviour management advice to families with children whose learning disability is complicated by behavioural difficulties
- teaching, training and consultation with staff working in special schools catering for children with learning disability
- input into the assessment and management of children with ASD
- consultation with social services personnel concerning their provision for families of children with a learning disability who also have mental health problems

- involvement in multi-agency learning disabilities services by liaison with staff such as paediatricians, educational psychologists, social workers, school doctors, etc.
- teaching and training to other agencies involved with children with a learning disability
- the development of close links with adult learning disability services
- presentations, discussions and liaison with parent support groups
- family therapy
- audit of team performance
- organisation and running of groups for children (e.g. social skills groups).

Assessment process

Families with children with learning disabilities present with a wide range of complex problems. Comprehensive assessment, including of the school and home environment, is vital before a formulation and intervention plan can be made. The American Association for Mental Retardation (1992) provides a useful framework for assessment (Table 19.1).

Joint assessments with professionals at child development centres should be considered for children with complex problems where there is a mental health component.

Table 19.1 Diagnostic protocol (American Association on Mental Retardation, 1992, with permission)

Dimension	Assessment
Dimension I: intellectual functioning and adaptive skills	There are a number of standardised psychological tests for assessing intellectual ability – e.g. the Griffiths Mental Developmental Scales from Birth (Huntley, 1996), British Ability Scales (Elliot 1996), Wechsler Intelligence Scale for Children (3rd edn) (WISC III) (Wechsler, 1991) – and adaptive behaviour, e.g. Vineland Adaptive Behavior Scales (Sparrow *et al*, 1984)
Dimension II: psychological and emotional status	Assessed by clinical interview, observation and behaviour scales, e.g. Child Behaviour Checklist (Achenbach, 1991)
Dimension III: physical, health and aetiological factors	Usually assessed by paediatricians
Dimension IV: environmental factors	

Intervention

A mental health service for children with a learning disability and their families should be able to offer:

- information – giving parents clear, unambiguous information about the child's disability and the implications of the diagnosis
- counselling – helping the family to deal with their emotional distress on diagnosis and at transitional periods in the child's life
- support – providing clear information about available support systems, such as respite services, portage, parents' support groups
- referral to other services, such as paediatrics, speech therapists, pre-school teaching services, social services, where indicated
- behavioural management – functional analysis and assessment of patterns of behaviours (Oliver, 1995) and the development of effective strategies and support with and for parents
- individual or group sessions to help children to develop a variety of life skills
- family therapy
- medication.

Consultation and liaison

Consultation and liaison with professionals working directly with children with learning disabilities and their families is an integral part of the work of a CAMHS learning disabilities team. Children will often be known to several agencies. Regular discussion between professionals is essential in coordinating services, avoiding duplication of work and establishing consistency of approaches. Formal meetings or forums are often generated by commonality of symptomatology or intervention programmes for disorders such as ASD or attentional problems. Similarly, it may be helpful to form a multi-agency learning disabilities team, which could meet monthly or bi-monthly to discuss children with complex needs. One of the members of the team should take responsibility for compiling a list of children to be discussed, at the request of team members, and circulating this before meetings.

Establishing relationships with staff in special schools and respite care services should be considered as a major role for a CAMHS learning disabilities team. A regular presence, possibly once each term, allows the opportunity for informal discussion and early intervention.

Transition from child to adult services

The transition from child to adult services is a particularly significant time for young people with learning disabilities. Many changes happen simultaneously, making this time especially stressful for them and their families. This transitional period should be carefully managed. However, some of the literature suggests that this is not usually the case (Tutt, 1995). Families report a host of dilemmas (Thorin *et al*, 1996), with which they would value help and support. Examples include learning to cope with the changes and losses, and wanting to create opportunities for independence while assuring that health and safety needs are met. Ideally, the planning process should be part of on-going therapeutic interventions, with a more formal process occurring when the young person is around 14 years of age. Some areas have a policy of organising multi-agency meetings with families as part of the school review. The personal and sensitive transfer of care should ease the transition from child to adult services.

Teaching and training

When working in a specialist area it is important to disseminate information at all opportunities. Information about different types of syndromes and intellectual disabilities can be shared with staff in schools and colleges, social services and voluntary agencies, as well as with parent support groups, in order to encourage understanding, early detection and intervention strategies. Staff in special schools often value workshops related to the management of challenging behaviours.

Evaluation

To ensure the service is effective, it must have clear objectives and an operational policy that is directed to meeting those objectives. Audit and the collection of user perspectives are the methods by which the service is monitored and developed.

Audit

The service should be audited at least yearly, in order to monitor referral rates, presenting problems, assessment protocols and interventions. Such audits (Green *et al*, 2001) establish whether the standards set for the service are being maintained, but also demonstrate where future challenges for the service may lie, for example if referral rates far exceed discharge rates.

User perspectives

The service offered should not only meet the needs of children with learning disabilities and their families, but also be provided in a manner they find acceptable and supportive. Attendance at parent support groups can help to provide insight into perceptions and offer a foundation for the development of user surveys. Awareness of the strengths and weaknesses of the service allows for re-evaluation and change. Similarly, professionals working with and using the service can offer important insights into the development of the team.

Conclusion

Children with learning disabilities who also have mental disorders and mental health problems have specific needs, as do their families. If services are expected to be delivered by generic CAMHS or 'life span' learning disabilities services, these specific needs are likely to be ill understood and poorly met. If the objectives of *Valuing People* (Department of Health, 2001c) are truly to be met in children and young people, specialised services with specially trained staff are required.

CHAPTER 20

Autistic spectrum disorders services

Christine Williams and Barry Wright

'The NAS [National Autistic Society] holds that there is an unacceptable gap between Learning Disability services for those with an IQ of less than 70, and Mental Health services into which a large number of people with an Autistic Spectrum Disorder are currently falling ... individuals with autism and in particular, Asperger's syndrome are commonly misdiagnosed, with medication inappropriately prescribed. The current system of NHS Mental Health provision, is therefore failing a minority of people with Autistic Spectrum Disorder, who may go on to present severely anti-social or self-destructive behaviour, resulting in admission to Mental Health services, Special Hospitals or prison services.'
National Autistic Society (1983)

Introduction

Autistic spectrum disorders (ASD) are thought to affect many more people than is generally recognised. The most recent reviews indicate approximately 60 per 10 000 children under the age of eight years are affected (Medical Research Council, 2001).

Children and adolescents with ASD show abnormalities in:

- communication and language development
- reciprocal social interaction
- symbolic play
- patterns of interests (the range of interests is restricted, and they centre on repetitive or stereotyped activities).

A number of different disorders appear to overlap, each overlapping disorder having different characteristics (Figure 20.1).

Difficulties in each of these areas vary considerably in both severity and the combination of factors. The autistic spectrum includes the syndromes described by Kanner (1943) and by Asperger (1944) but is wider than these two subgroups (Wing & Gould, 1979). CAMHS are frequently asked to assess children who may have ASD and such assessment is fraught with difficulties, as described in Box 20.1.

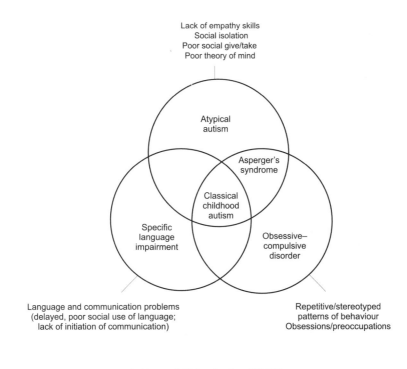

Lack of empathy skills
Social isolation
Poor social give/take
Poor theory of mind

Atypical
autism

Asperger's
syndrome

Classical
childhood
autism

Specific
language
impairment

Obsessive–
compulsive
disorder

Language and communication problems
(delayed, poor social use of language;
lack of initiation of communication)

Repetitive/stereotyped
patterns of behaviour
Obsessions/preoccupations

Incidence of childhood autism: 4/10 000
Incidence of autistic spectrum disorders: 35/10 000

Figure 20.1 Overlap of disorders in connection with autism.

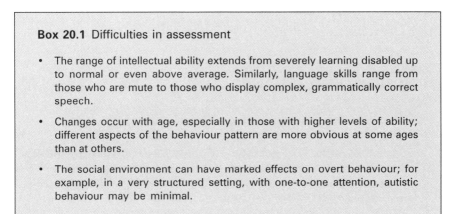

Box 20.1 Difficulties in assessment

- The range of intellectual ability extends from severely learning disabled up to normal or even above average. Similarly, language skills range from those who are mute to those who display complex, grammatically correct speech.

- Changes occur with age, especially in those with higher levels of ability; different aspects of the behaviour pattern are more obvious at some ages than at others.

- The social environment can have marked effects on overt behaviour; for example, in a very structured setting, with one-to-one attention, autistic behaviour may be minimal.

The organisation of assessment

There are various models for assessment. A clinical psychologist or a child psychiatrist would usually carry out an assessment within a CAMHS, but other professionals, such as paediatricians or speech and language therapists, should link to such assessments according to the models listed in Box 20.2.

Whichever model is used, assessment should be multi-disciplinary (Sparrow, 1997) and systematised to a protocol agreed between the different professionals involved. There should be a core diagnostic team of paediatrician, child psychiatrist, clinical psychologist and speech therapist with access to additional professionals, including the child's teacher, educational psychologist, learning support teacher or special educational needs coordinator. Other professionals who may be called upon to be involved in the assessment include social workers, family workers, occupational therapists, physiotherapists, school doctors, school nurses, autism specialist workers, community psychiatric nurses, portage workers and respite care workers.

When parents become aware of, or are alerted to, their child's abnormal development, they are usually referred to a consultant community paediatrician, who assesses the child and, on the basis of examination and investigations, will form an opinion about the child's difficulties. Sometimes the child is referred to a member of the CAMHS, particularly if he or she is older and of normal IQ with, for example, Asperger's syndrome.

Whatever the route, there should be a strong emphasis on the partnership between parents and professionals throughout. Information about the content and process of assessment and diagnosis should be shared and discussed openly. There should be no surprises when a final diagnosis is made, as parents should be given a clear rationale and justification for the clinician's formulation throughout the procedure. This allows for the building of a trusting relationship, which is vital in

---

Box 20.2 Models of assessment

- A child psychiatrist, clinical psychologist or both linking to a full team, or comprehensive assessment arranged in a child development centre.
- Each professional carrying out their own assessment in their own clinic, but having mechanisms to discuss and coordinate information, and arrive at mutually agreed decisions about diagnosis and management
- A specifically arranged assessment process (either ad hoc or systematised) that coordinates assessment between clinicians, and allows for co-ordinated diagnostic formulation and management plans.

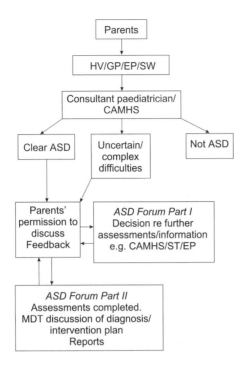

Figure 20.2 Protocol for an autistic spectrum disorders (ASD) forum. EP, educational psychologist; HV, health visitor; MDT, multi-disciplinary team; SW, social worker; ST, support teacher.

helping parents to make sense of their child's difficulties, their own emotional distress and intervention strategies.

If autistic symptoms are unclear or the clinician is uncertain, the child may be referred to a multi-disciplinary forum involving those working with these children, with the parents' consent, to clarify the diagnosis or to discuss management strategies. A protocol for the organisation of referral for assessment and the usage of such a forum is detailed in Figure 20.2.

Such a forum would be held at regular intervals, perhaps bimonthly. In the first part of the meeting, children who are being presented for the first time are discussed. Decisions about further assessments and information to be gathered are made in relation to:

- history
- autistic symptoms
- observation
- paediatric assessment
- cognitive/developmental assessment

- speech and language assessment
- occupational therapy assessment, including fine and gross motor skills
- physiotherapy assessment, including self-help skills and physical functioning
- social services assessment for service provision
- consideration of alternative diagnoses, such as hearing impairment, learning disability, developmental language delay or severe psychosocial deprivation.

With parents' permission, these assessments are completed before the next forum.

In the second part of the forum, children whose assessments have been completed are discussed and a diagnosis is made, if indicated. Occasionally, a decision to defer a diagnosis may be made on the basis of uncertainty about the extent to which other factors (e.g. hearing loss, severe language impairment, or global developmental delay) may account for the symptoms. In this case another date will be set for review.

Discussion about appropriate, available interventions from each agency should follow. This should be detailed in the final report on the child and offered to the child's parents, with an opportunity for discussion so that they can correct any points of fact and ask any further questions. The final copy should then be sent back to the parents and other professionals to whom it is relevant.

Establishing a service for children with autistic spectrum disorder

In some CAMHS, ASD fall within the remit of a learning disabilities team, in view of the considerable overlap of the two populations. However, this is a discrete subgroup of children who may justify their own Tier 3 team within CAMHS. Such specialist provision has the following the advantages:

- clarity of purpose
- networking of professionals working collaboratively to the benefit of children and families
- the opportunity to generate an identity (e.g. with a name such as autistic spectrum disorders forum) that encourages the development of expertise and cooperative working
- it facilitates the development of a policy and protocol for working, based around procedures for assessing, making diagnoses and formulating/coordinating management plans
- the development of a common language and nomenclature across agencies and disciplines

- the operation of common diagnostic procedures
- joined-up thinking in the planning of interventions
- clear inter-agency planning of services for children and young people with ASD
- efficiency
- improved user and carer experiences.

The establishment of such a team then provides a focus for the development of a strategy to deliver services to children with ASD and their families.

Screening

The possibility of systematising screening for ASD into health visitor or general practitioner developmental checks should be encouraged by CAMHS. For example, the Checklist for Autism in Toddlers (CHAT; Baron-Cohen *et al*, 1992) is an early screening tool that may be used at the 18-month check; it has been found useful for primary care professionals, particularly health visitors, who have regular access to under-fives. The service should then allow those working at Tier 1 access to Tier 2 professionals, who are experienced at working with these children and families, and to Tier 3 teams such as an ASD team. Many professionals such as teachers may have concerns about a child's socialisation or communication skills, for instance, without necessarily being aware of some of the features of ASD, particularly at the milder end of the spectrum. They need to have access to consultation and referral. In some teams this may be systematised in, for example, formal consultation sessions with health visitors, school nurses or paediatric liaison teams.

Training

The National Autistic Society estimates that ASD are greatly under-diagnosed. It recommends that health professionals be trained in developing awareness of symptoms. Paediatricians and CAMHS with expertise in these areas are encouraged to help to build understanding of ASD within Tier 1 by supplying information and running workshops.

Training must also emphasise basic topics such as confidentiality, parental consent and ways of sharing concerns about young people with parents. These are issues that can be forgotten when dealing with children with poor communication skills.

Professionals engaged in the assessment and diagnosis of children with ASD should ensure that their skills are up to date by attendance at one of the courses available to them. Such courses include training in the use of the Diagnostic Interview for Social and Communication Disorders (DISCO) (Leekam *et al*, 2002; Wing *et al*, 2002), the Autism Diagnostic Interview – Revised (ADI–R; Lord *et al*, 1994) and the Autism Diagnostic Observation Schedule – Generic (ADOS-G; Lord *et al*, 2000).

Interventions

There is no known cure for autism (Cohen & Volkmar, 1997). Intervention is based on helping children to develop strategies to compensate for their difficulties with communication, preventing secondary emotional dysfunction and helping parents to manage their children's behaviour in order that they may all lead as normal a life as possible. It is good practice for intervention to begin at first contact with parents; shared goals should be agreed and a partnership established. This should continue throughout the assessment and treatment process. A comprehensive intervention programme involves the following:

- Information about ASD – providing the family with information about assessment, diagnosis and prognosis. This can occur throughout the assessment process through general discussion and by giving information sheets. The National Autistic Society (NAS) provides a wide range of literature.
- Information about local services, including:
  - parent support groups
  - groups for young people with ASD
  - individual therapeutic work for children with ASD
  - computer-based instruction (Williams *et al*, 2003)
  - respite services
  - Crossroads Association
  - portage
  - social services facilities
  - education services
  - Sure Start
  - autism workers.
- Educational placement – the educational psychologist should take responsibility for guiding parents through the options available locally.
- Family support – many families benefit from the availability of support to help them to understand and cope with the grief process that often follows diagnosis.
- Strategies for managing behaviour.
- TEACHH (Schopler, 1997) – a structured learning programme aimed at utilising the strengths of children with ASD.

- Behaviourally based treatment strategies (e.g. Lovaas, 1987).
- Medication.
- Parent training intervention packages.
- Early Bird (National Autistic Society).
- Adapted Haven Programme.
- Help with the transition from child and adolescent services to adult services. This can be a particularly stressful period for families and requires careful liaison between the professionals working in the two services.

Conclusion

Children with ASD are recognised at different stages of their lives. Autism is often recognised early, whereas Asperger's syndrome may not be recognised until adolescence. Sensitivity to the possibility of the diagnosis must be present in all those who work with children and young people at all developmental stages so that assessment of their complex needs is competently undertaken and management strategies instituted in all areas of the child's functioning.

CHAPTER 21

Attentional problems services

Barry Wright and Christine Williams

'I always keep a supply of stimulant handy in case I see a snake – which I also keep handy.'
W. C. Fields

Introduction

CAMHS are regularly called upon to assess children who have problems with attention, concentration, distractibility, impulsiveness, over-activity or a combination of these. These difficulties may be part of attention-deficit hyperactivity disorder (ADHD) or may be symptoms of other problems. ADHD is a condition where the symptom profile and aetiology are regularly being redefined. Recent reviews outline some of the research driving current thinking (Overmeyer & Taylor, 1999; Williams *et al*, 1999*b*). Recent guidelines from the National Institute for Clinical Excellence and a large American study (MTA Cooperative Group, 1999) have also informed good practice. As additional resources have often not generally been forthcoming to support such good practice, existing services may restructure aspects of their functioning in order to form Tier 3 teams.

One way of rationalising resources effectively is to establish inter-agency links so that multi-disciplinary working is not limited by professional boundaries. Some centres have done just this to meet the needs of children with complex problems, including ADHD complicated by comorbid difficulties (Williams *et al*, 1999*b*). Where there is no coordinated approach to assessment and intervention for children who present with these difficulties, confusion may arise and contradictory advice may be given by different agencies. Parents and carers need to feel confident that professionals are working with them and with other agencies to provide a comprehensive assessment and treatment package for their children. A Tier 3 team within a CAMHS has the advantage of multi-disciplinary working, and this facilitates the development of shared learning and understanding, and the evolution of clear protocols (Voeller, 1991). A specific attentional problems clinic can provide assessment, diagnosis, monitoring and a range of on-going interventions.

Box 21.1 Principles of service provision

- Multi-disciplinary working.
- A clear operational policy.
- A responsive service with good feedback to the referrer.
- A protocol for assessment and diagnosis that is regularly audited.
- A range of interventions that takes on the social, educational, emotional and medical needs of the young person and family.
- A cooperative alliance with families.
- A protocol for communication with education services.
- Information to other services about routes of consultation and referral.

The attentional problems team should ideally include a child psychiatrist, a clinical psychologist and a community psychiatric nurse. The service will be enhanced by input from other CAMHS team members, such as occupational therapists, social workers or social services family workers, education support staff, and members of the child health team, for example community paediatricians, school doctors and school nurses. The principles of the team's service provision are set out in Box 21.1.

Many conditions and life situations can create problems with attention and concentration (Orford, 1998) and it is important to bear this in mind when assessing children with attentional problems.

An important managerial task is to ensure that a thorough assessment has taken place, that the formulation of the child's problems takes all relevant factors into consideration (and does not become linear) and that interventions seek to address the formulation rather than focusing exclusively on medication.

The nature of the service

In different centres, different professionals or teams carry out assessment. For example, community or hospital paediatricians may be involved in assessment and diagnosis. This works well when integrated with CAMHS. Many paediatric teams work closely with child mental health teams (Bingley et al, 1980; Dungar et al, 1986; Black et al, 1999) and the paediatrician may be linked to a CAMHS through joint clinics or meetings (Voeller, 1991). In this way, if paediatricians are making the diagnosis, they may be part of a multi-disciplinary service that assesses, diagnoses and formulates treatment plans based on a protocol that reflects shared beliefs about appropriate practice worked out in a coordinated fashion.

Cooperative working with CAMHS aside, the service can also be provided by the child development centre or as part of paediatric services, where professionals such as clinical psychologists and community nurses are employed within the team and can deliver a range of interventions. With either of these ways of working, it is still appropriate to make links with education support staff.

If a paediatric unit has stand-alone diagnostic and treatment services, this does not create difficulties if a full range of options is open to children and families. Problems may arise if treatment options are restricted. Some diagnosing paediatricians provide medication and ask the CAMHS to provide psychosocial interventions for children with ADHD but without granting the CAMHS any input to the assessment process. This may be problematic to the CAMHS, particularly if assessment standards that it sets for itself are not being met by the diagnosing service. Moreover, interventions are best planned during assessment, as there is a need to influence (before diagnosis) early attributions about the meaning of ADHD for the child and the family. Such attributions have an impact on how parents manage their child, what treatments are acceptable to families and what beliefs are passed on to the child (Wright et al, 2000). All these are likely to influence prognosis. In addition, since diagnosis is there to clarify and facilitate management possibilities, it makes no sense to divorce the two. Most CAMHS believe in either unified services, where one team or another has full responsibility for assessment, diagnosis and the full range of interventions, or integrated services where both child health services and child mental health services work closely together. Split services, where one service is expected to make diagnoses and the other to provide the bulk of the management, present incoherent practice to children and their carers. What these issues point to is a clear need for CAMHS and child health services to discuss roles and responsibilities with respect to these children and to have clear and agreed ways of working with each other. This is especially the case when second opinions are sought, as a second opinion must be integrated into the local management package (Richardson & Cottrell, 2003).

Assessment

Figure 21.1 outlines a protocol for the assessment of children with attentional problems. First, a detailed history and thorough assessment are, as always, essential. The time spent during this process not only provides valuable information but also facilitates the building of a relationship with the family. Parents should be consulted throughout the assessment process, and be allowed to ask questions and seek clarification. Questionnaires from home and school are helpful (Barkley,

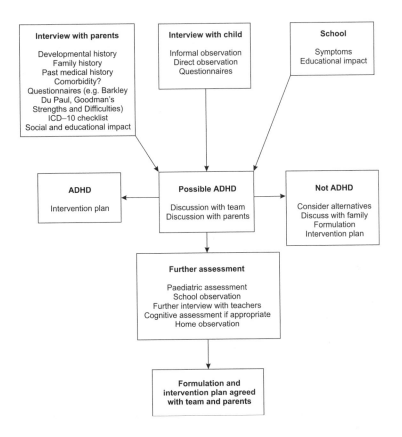

Figure 21.1 Protocol for ADHD assessment of children aged five years and over.

1990; Goodman, 2001). Clinicians should be mindful of the family's attributions about the child's difficulties, as these will have important implications for intervention. For example, if parents believe that the child's attentional and behavioural difficulties are entirely related to a biological problem requiring only medication as the remedy, they may be reluctant to engage in additional treatment programmes aimed at empowering both the child and parents (Wright *et al*, 2000).

If the team is sure that the child does not have ADHD, the family should be given clear information about their reason for this and alternative explanations for the child's behaviour should be discussed in detail. If ADHD cannot be ruled out at this stage, further investigations should be carried out, including a paediatric assessment, direct observations at school, interviews with teachers and an educational psychology assessment, if indicated. If a cognitive assessment has not already been completed and the child is on stage 4 or 5 of the educational special needs register, it may be helpful to make a referral for this purpose. An educational psychologist would usually carry out this work. This often provides important information about the child's intellectual ability, strengths, weaknesses and discrepancies.

When the information has been gathered, a formulation can be agreed with the team and the family. This should take into account the often complex interactions between physiological, psychological, developmental and psychosocial factors which assessment may have highlighted. Good liaison and communication with all agencies help to facilitate a joint understanding and hence a strong supported intervention plan.

Intervention

Given the varied options for treatment and on-going research, it is sensible for services to establish standards for the treatment of ADHD that can be regularly audited and reviewed.

- Children should have gone through a clear assessment protocol (see Figure 21.1) before intervention packages are discussed with families.
- Multi-faceted (psychosocial and educational) intervention packages should be tested.
- There should be clear monitoring of interventions both at home and at school, using narratives and questionnaires.
- Criteria for the use of medication should be established, based on factors such as age, severity and pervasiveness of symptoms and response to psychosocial interventions. Clear diagnosis of ADHD (or hyperkinetic disorder) must be established, for example by Research Diagnostic Criteria, and the condition should be seriously affecting social and educational functioning.
- Family attributions about the illness need to be considered and addressed to avoid attributions that militate against a better prognosis, or hamper healthy beliefs about medication.

Where medication is considered appropriate (Joughin & Zwi, 1999), the following are required:

- compliance with national guidelines (National Institute for Clinical Excellence, 2000)
- clear liaison with school (with parental permission) to establish a protocol for giving the child the medication in school if required and keeping it safely locked up (leaflet to school)
- checking of cautions and contraindications

- a protocol to establish a trial of medication (e.g. over a four-week period) with monitoring (e.g. by questionnaire) at home and particularly at school
- baseline information and information during and after the trial, including weight, height, blood pressure readings, pulse, narrative information from parents and teachers and questionnaires from teachers and parents
- liaison to keep the general practitioner informed (usually by letter) and to establish repeat prescribing according to local custom
- a protocol for the establishment of drug holidays (weekdays or school holidays or annually, as appropriate), to avoid the theoretical risk of disturbance of growth patterns and to assess symptom pattern changes with and without medication as the young person develops
- on-going monitoring, with clear plans agreed and reviews at agreed time points
- on-going psychosocial and educational interventions.

Intervention should be tailored to the child and family's needs, and strong links between all agencies must be maintained. The research literature suggests that single-treatment approaches (e.g. either medication or behavioural modification) have several shortcomings. Pelham *et al* (1993) found that these could be reduced when approaches are combined, with suggestions that the primary symptoms are most successfully treated by medication and the secondary symptoms by behavioural approaches. The large MTA Cooperative study in America suggests that improvement in most ADHD symptoms is obtained by medication alone, and is not enhanced by psychosocial interventions (MTA Cooperative Group, 1999). However, allied behaviour/conduct problems, social skills, internalising symptoms and reading achievement are all enhanced by psychosocial interventions (MTA Cooperative Group, 1999). More careful analysis of the data shows that childhood outcome from psychosocial interventions is clearest where process outcome is achieved, such as a reduction in negative, ineffective parenting (Hinshaw *et al*, 2000).

Box 21.2 summarises the treatment approaches.

Conclusion

ADHD teams usefully link paediatricians, child mental health professionals and professionals from education support services. The advantages of forming such a team include: the development of expertise and cooperative working; the facilitation of a protocol for assessment

Box 21.2 Treatment approaches

- Behaviour therapy and parenting programmes, whether large-scale and community based (Cunningham *et al*, 1995) or small-scale and focused (Overmeyer & Taylor, 1999), can reduce conduct problems in such children. Large-scale studies have confirmed this (MTA Cooperative Group, 1999).

- Individual work can include cognitive therapy (Whalen *et al*, 1985), aimed at helping children internalise external messages of control and social problem-solving skills training.

- Group work can focus on social skills (Pelham & Bender, 1982), social problem-solving skills or anger management skills. The MTA study included a summer treatment programme (Wells *et al*, 2001).

- Educational interventions enhance learning (Cantwell & Baker, 1992; Wells *et al*, 2001).

- Work on child and family attributions is also important. Unnecessary blame alienates families (Bramble, 1998) and other strategies may help to empower parents to manage children and to view themselves as part of a solution, and to allow the child to believe in the possibilities of positive change and self-control (Wright *et al*, 2000). In this way managing the attributions also becomes important in order to encourage healthy developmental trajectories for children.

- There is clear evidence that medication improves the concentration and reduces distractibility in most children, and therefore has clear benefits for children with ADHD in the short term (MTA Cooperative Group, 1999). Longer-term benefits are less well established and need to be further researched.

and diagnosis; and the coordination of management plans. Working with education services in particular helps to build a joint understanding which can be passed on to the teaching staff who have daily direct contact with the children.

CHAPTER 22

Eating disorders services

Ian Partridge and Greg Richardson

'How disenchanting in the female character is a manifestation of relish for the pleasures of the table!'
William Charles Macready

Introduction

Eating disorders are the subject of many debates with regard to both aetiology and treatment (Royal College of Psychiatrists, 1992a; Ward *et al*, 1995; Shoebridge & Gowers, 2000; Gowers & Shore, 2001), but the referral of young persons suffering from them to CAMHS is a constant. Specialist services for these young people are few (Lemouchoux *et al*, 2001). The establishment of a specialist service within a CAMHS is practicable and efficient. Such a service represents an optimal use of resources, in terms of both personnel and time (Roberts *et al*, 1998), and is effective (Schmidt, 2001). The principles that must underpin the service are set out in Box 22.1.

A specialist service integrated with locality CAMHS

Recently there has been a move towards the establishment of discrete eating disorders services as a response to consumer pressure and a perception by certain providers that such services are income generators.

Box 22.1 Service principles

- A multi-disciplinary approach.
- A clear operational policy.
- Prompt responses.
- A range of interventions geared to the individual needs of the young person and family.
- A continuum of care between out-patient and in-patient services.

There are none the less advantages to having a specialist eating disorders team operating within rather than without an existing CAMHS:

- It facilitates the coordinated utilisation of existing resources of personnel and time to provide a discrete and recognisable service.
- The models of treatment can be informed from a multi-disciplinary perspective.
- There is cohesion within the wider CAMHS, and specialist expertise and experience are not hived off and isolated, which avoids fragmentation of services and a blinkered team outlook. Specialist resources within a comprehensive CAMHS encourage the recognition that eating disorders often exist within a wider clinical context and may be concomitant with other psychological or psychiatric dysfunction.
- Team members can develop expertise that can be used to meet the training needs of a range of disciplines; training programmes can be offered to allied disciplines and, in consultation, to other agencies.
- The team can offer a range of treatment options while ensuring effective use of time so that individuals are seen speedily and regularly within the structure of a mutually supportive team. Supervision is built into the organisation of the team and can, if and when necessary, be live.
- The team may deal with the full age range, managing childhood-onset eating problems (Fox & Joughin, 2002) as well as anorexia and bulimia nervosa.
- The problem of differential funding for different disorders, with consequent inequity of access, is avoided. Those who put money making above the comprehensive and integrated care of populations may consider this a disadvantage.
- There may be fewer in-patient admissions (Richardson *et al*, 1998).
- A specific clinic whose purpose is well explained appears to reduce non-attendance rates and, as non-attendance can prove costly in terms of the allocation of team time, this improves efficiency.

Specialist provision within an existing CAMHS is labour intensive and removes resources from existing service provision; however, these young people would still have to be managed by the service. Pressure upon such a small service could lead to the lengthening of waiting lists, but if the team is of sufficient size and clinics operate for sufficient sessions per week to meet the demands of the catchment population, this should not be a problem. The team then provides an initial assessment service as well as a variety of ongoing therapeutic interventions from various permutations of the team working individually and jointly. Flexibility may entail occasional working outside of the structured sessional timetable.

Referral and intervention

A specialist eating disorders team may receive referrals direct from the allocation process, as well as from other members of the CAMHS. The eating disorders team can discuss all referrals, prioritise them and allocate them to specific professionals. A standardised, explanatory appointment letter should be sent to the young person and family with an offer of an appointment within four weeks of referral. There may need to be emergency responses to acute crises. At the initial assessment (see Box 22.2) the whole family should be asked to attend so that from the start there is a clear message that the family is the most powerful therapeutic tool currently available for adolescents (Russell *et al*, 1987).

An initial management plan is negotiated with the family; this plan must take into account developmental, physical and psychological considerations. The possible physical consequences of eating disorders may dictate medical treatment and therefore the team should be keen to establish close working relationships with colleagues in paediatrics, endocrinology and gastroenterological medicine.

The team should offer a range of therapeutic options, including advice on management, often based on behavioural principles, cognitive–behavioural therapy (Schmidt, 1998), motivational interviewing (Treasure & Schmidt, 2001), guided reading (Schmidt & Treasure, 1993), family therapy (Russell *et al*, 1987) and, if absolutely necessary, in-patient treatment. Factors that influence the need for in-patient care include:

- weight loss of more than 25% or a body mass index (BMI) of less than 13
- refusal of all food and drink (dehydration being of major concern)
- rehabilitation after medical admission because of the physical consequences of the eating disorder
- the young person's specific request for in-patient care
- failure of prolonged out-patient treatment.

Box 22.2 Assessment protocol

- History of presenting problem and update on present situation.
- Physical examination and investigation, including height and weight.
- Questionnaires such as the Eating Attitude Test (EAT).
- Full family, medical and psychiatric histories.
- Interview with parents.
- Interview with child.

The aim of in-patient care of anorexia nervosa is to return the young person to developmentally appropriate physical and psychological functioning through weight gain, but there is a worse prognosis for young people who are admitted (Gowers *et al*, 2000), which may reflect the more serious nature of their condition.

Conclusion

Eating disorders present complex bio-psychosocial difficulties to the sufferers, their carers and involved professionals. These are likely to be alleviated only by work from many perspectives that is geared to supporting the young person and family in developing eating patterns that ensure health; it is necessary to facilitate the addressing of issues that may be being avoided by the individual and the family through the mechanism of the eating disorder.

CHAPTER 23

Bereavement services

Barry Wright and Ian Partridge

'To the bereaved nothing but the return of the lost person can bring true comfort; should what we provide fall short of that it is felt almost as an insult.'
John Bowlby

Introduction

Bereavement is not a pathological process. Although some children may suffer significant psychological consequences (Pettle-Michael & Lansdown, 1986), depression is rare (Pfeffer *et al*, 2000). The evidence for the efficacy or usefulness of therapeutic work is limited (Harrington & Harrison, 1999).

Indications for bereavement work

Children may need support at times of family bereavement. There are a number of reasons why the impact of bereavement on the development of children can be marked:

- the bereavement may be associated with circumstances in which the normal supportive family influences are severely hampered; such circumstances include parental mental illness (Van Eerdewegh *et al*, 1985), catastrophic parental bereavement responses, and emotionally abusive or neglecting parents (Elizur & Kaffman, 1983; Bifulco *et al*, 1987)
- there may be severe psychological trauma associated with the death, including parental suicide (Wright & Partridge, 1999; Pfeffer *et al*, 2000)
- a child may suffer repeated bereavement
- a bereavement may result in prolonged disruption to the child's life
- bereavement may bring about family system changes (Wasserman, 1988)
- extreme circumstances, such as war (Goldstein *et al*, 1997).

Box 23.1 Functions of bereavement team

- Treating mental health problems in the child.
- Prevention of child mental ill health by working with children at high risk.
- Prevention of future child mental ill health by working with parents, including preventing mental ill health in a parent.
- Leadership and consultation in fashioning district-wide services, and coordinating and integrating statutory and voluntary agencies in their provision.

Managing bereavement

Childhood bereavement services look at the effects of bereavement on children in a number of ways:

- *Diagnostically*. Bereavement can lead to emotional or behavioural problems that have social or educational effects and that represent a diagnosable entity.
- *Adult mental health*. There may be effects on the parenting available to the child before or after the bereavement.
- *Child protection*. A bereavement may upset parents' emotional or physical care of a child.
- *Systemically*. There may be systemic effects that represent risk factors for the child.
- *Developmentally*. The circumstances surrounding the bereavement may damage the child's development.
- *Attributionally*. Beliefs and attributions regarding the death, in either the child or the family, may be damaging.

In considering these factors, the CAMHS needs to have a clear view of its functions (Box 23.1).

There appears to be a spectrum of provision throughout the country, ranging from CAMHS that have no involvement with bereavement unless a diagnosable mental disorder is present, to CAMHS that take a lead role in coordinating, and integrating with, a range of bereavement services across a district.

In practice, CAMHS can be usefully involved in:

- networking with other professionals to ensure a comprehensive range of services
- providing consultation to those supporting children and their families (such as teachers, general practice counsellors, school

nurses, Cruse counsellors, pupil support staff, social workers, family support workers, general practitioners and chaplains)

- taking referrals for those bereaved children with emotional and behavioural problems where families and Tier 1 professionals are struggling.

Networking

Parents or carers are best placed to support bereaved children, although they may call on Tier 1 professionals for support. The involvement of Tier 2 professionals may occur subsequently if there are clear indications of a mental health problem.

It is common sense for the various professionals involved in bereavement support to know each other and to have an understanding of the way services relate to each other. There are a number of ways to achieve this, including networking meetings or established mechanisms for liaison. Formal links may be usefully established through:

- palliative care teams
- local adult hospices
- local children's hospices
- Cruse counsellors
- health visitors
- school nurses
- hospital chaplaincy services
- pupil support services.

Such links serve to highlight existing services and gaps in services that the network may decide to address. The tasks will include offering advice and support in a family-centred provision that dovetails with services from other agencies; key aims must be to avoid both stigma and the disempowering of families.

CAMHS have an important advice and consultation role, and may be able to draw upon a range of models to inform, advise and support. Team members will be able to draw on their understanding of the following:

- attachment issues (Bowlby, 1980) that acknowledge a young person's fear of rejection, isolation, not being understood, or fears for the future (Balk, 1990; Silverman et al, 1992)
- systemic issues, including changes in roles within the family, and changes in affective functioning within the family (Wasserman, 1988)
- how children may experience significant psychological and behavioural difficulties in bereavement (Pettle-Michael & Lansdown, 1986)

- communication and how adult anxiety may affect healthy coping (Baulkwill & Wood, 1994)
- the importance of maintaining family integrity and self-efficacy (Bandura *et al*, 1980; Silverman & Worden, 1992)
- the child's age and developmental stage (Kane, 1979)
- the importance of establishing the meaning of events to the child (Pollock, 1986)
- adjustment as family members simultaneously negotiate change (Silverman *et al*, 1992)
- the factors other than bereavement that may affect a child, and the need to arrive at a formulation that takes account of emotional, psychosocial, intellectual, educational, developmental, family and environmental factors
- that bereavement in itself is not a pathological process, although a range of vulnerability factors and resilience factors may be operating at both the parental (e.g. poor parenting after the death of one parent, parental mental illness) and the child level (e.g. social and peer support, intelligence) that can have an effect on both present and future child mental health.

Team membership

While all CAMHS members would normally be expected to have a grasp of issues relating to bereavement, and to be able to provide consultation and take referrals where necessary, there may be a number of reasons to identify certain professionals within the team to take a lead role with bereavement:

- to enable them to develop more expertise in particularly difficult scenarios such as suicide
- to provide a focus for consultation and liaison with other teams (palliative care, hospices, paediatric liaison, etc.)
- to take a lead role in networking
- to take a lead role in the development of services.

Any of the professionals within the CAMHS would be able to do this. In larger areas, two or more professionals may share this work. Formal referrals can be processed through the allocation process.

Planning and training

CAMHS members may need training from time to time in this area, since such referrals are not uncommon. By the same token, CAMHS professionals may be called on to provide training for a variety of other professionals, from both voluntary and statutory agencies.

Box 23.2 Possible interventions

- Provision of information.
- Advice to parents, carers and other supporting adults.
- Consultation to Tier 1 professionals.
- Individual work.
- Group work (Pennels *et al*, 1992; Baulkwill & Wood, 1994; Smith & Pennels, 1995; Wright *et al*, 1996).
- Family work (Gibbons, 1992; Gillance *et al*, 1997).

Interventions

Clinicians would usually encourage good emotional and psychological support from the family, with open and honest communication with the child about the death. Few more specific interventions have been systematically studied (Harrington, 1998). Consideration needs to be given to the justification of any intervention in terms of the benefits for the child and family. Box 23.2 lists the interventions that a CAMHS may consider providing.

Multi-agency groups

In some districts the development of groups may involve professionals from different agencies (voluntary and statutory) coming together. In this way they bring children, with whom they may have been working individually, into a group setting. Since this can be set up in such a way as to involve the same number of hours of work, it can be resource neutral to each agency. This allows children to work alongside each other and means that no agency commits more time than it would have committed ordinarily. Groups do not preclude individual or family work before or after group work. This has the advantages of:

- providing a wider range of services for children and families
- improving professional networking
- cross-fertilisation of ideas among local professionals
- improving peer supervision
- avoiding stigmatisation engendered by referral to mental health services.

Once a networked service is established, it is necessary for professionals at Tier 1 to be aware both of its existence and of the range of services available. This can be done by providing relevant information to primary mental health link workers, general practice surgeries, customer service departments within social services, hospital chaplaincy, palliative care teams and pupil support services. Such information should include a service map that delineates all the various agencies, contact details, their expertise, how they work and how they relate to other professionals.

Audit and evaluation

Regular audit ensures that services have standards and maintain them. More research needs to be done to clarify the role of bereavement support services. Families should be asked for feedback about services and be given evaluation forms. It is necessary to ensure that services are accessible to all children and their families, including those with special needs (e.g. children with disabilities or sensory impairments).

CHAPTER 24

Drug and alcohol teams

Norman Malcolm

'Anxiety + Concerns + Heroin = No Problem'
Heroin user

Why we need substance misuse services

In the minds of both professionals and the public at large, substance use and subsequent misuse seem to have become ubiquitous. There have been other times when this was the case; however, there are now distinct differences, that include:

- declining age of initiation into substance use
- a steep rise in the use of heroin
- multiple drug use
- prevalence of use by girls approaching that of boys
- widespread availability of illicit substances
- proposed link between substance misuse and an increased rate of completed suicide for men aged 15–24 years
- widespread use of cannabis, stimulants and LSD within the dance/rave culture.

More young people than ever before are aware of psychoactive substances, know people who use them and use them themselves. The likelihood exists, therefore, of greater numbers of young people experiencing problems with substance use.

Not surprisingly, young people whose development has already been compromised by a variety of adverse life events may initially find solace in substance use and later find themselves compounding their problems when the negative effects begin to accrue. This has begun to show itself in the high levels of problematic substance use in at-risk groups, including:

- looked after children
- homeless young people
- children and young people who have experienced abuse
- school excludees
- children and young people from disrupted family backgrounds
- children and young people whose parents misuse substances.

CAMHS are being asked to join with colleagues in social services, education and the voluntary sector to provide services for the same young people featured in the list above. As they do so, it is clear that CAMHS will be working with young people who are misusing substances. As the 1996 thematic review of substance misuse services for children and young people (NHS Health Advisory Service, 1996) as well as the more recent 2001 review (NHS Health Advisory Service, 2001) have shown, existing provision is patchy; if it exists at all, it is often added on to adult services. Current thinking across the board is that services for young substance users must be child focused and take account of primary and secondary prevention as well as treatment. Government policy, as outlined in *Tackling Drugs to Build a Better Britain* (HM Government, 1998), emphasises the need for commissioners and providers of services to focus on young people as one of the four main priority areas for intervention. The response needs to be multi-disciplinary if it is to succeed in addressing the complex social problems that coexist with substance misuse. The specialist medical and therapeutic skills within CAMHS will be an essential element of an effective response.

Strategic planning process

As well as seeing patients, a specialist CAMHS substance misuse team will need to contribute to the strategic planning processes that currently exist (Box 24.1). Recent changes to strategic planning structures include the setting up of locality-based primary care trusts and the establishment on 1 April 2001 of the National Treatment Agency (NTA), a Special Health Authority within the National Health Service charged with increasing the capacity, quality and effectiveness of drug treatment in England – in its own words, ensuring the availability of 'More Treatment, Better Treatment and Fairer Treatment' (Paul Hayes, Chief Executive, National Treatment Agency).

Government targets with regard to drug misuse are laid out in the ten-year strategy that began in 1998 and drugs services for young

---

Box 24.1 National strategic planning structure

- Government ten-year strategy, *Tackling Drugs to Build a Better Britain*.
- National Treatment Agency (Chief Executive Paul Hayes).
- Nine regional NTA managers based in the Government Offices for the Regions.
- Home Office Drug Prevention and Advisory Service (DPAS).
- 150 drug action teams and drug and alcohol action teams.
- Drug and alcohol reference groups and task groups.

---

people are now a national priority. Although not required by law in England, around 50% of drug action teams (DATs) have now included alcohol misuse within their planning structures, and so have become drug and alcohol action teams (DAATs). The UK drugs strategy has the doubling of the availability of drug treatment as a key target. DAATs are responsible for coordinating a multi-agency response to meet the government's targets within the broad principles of integration, evidence, joint action, consistency, effective communication, quality standards and accountability. Local planning structures are required to contribute to strategic plans to meet the needs of young substance users and to report to government via the NTA.

Perhaps the two most relevant targets within the strategy for CAMHS to consider are:

• young people – to help young people resist drug misuse in order to achieve their full potential in society

• treatment – to enable individuals with drug problems to overcome them and live healthy and crime-free lives.

Local strategic planning structures and membership of relevant bodies will vary geographically, although the majority of such structures are likely to include task groups focusing on each of the four main target areas: young people, communities, treatment and availability. CAMHS should be represented on the groups addressing issues regarding young people and treatment. Whatever the local structure, DAATs should not work in isolation from, and neither should they be seen as replacing, existing planning structures for children and young people. There should be close collaboration between these bodies, which may include the Integrated Children's Services Plan, the Area Child Protection Committee, the Health Improvement Plan, and structures surrounding education, youth offending and the needs of minority ethnic groups. CAMHS may already be represented on some or all of the groups.

How the service responds

The setting up of a drug and alcohol team within a CAMHS, and subsequently with those with whom they form working partnerships, depends on finding those with an interest in and knowledge of substance misuse. This has obvious training and recruitment implications and there is wide geographical variation in this respect. Team membership therefore may be very varied in terms of professional disciplines and ultimately in the service they can provide.

Furthermore, there is variation in the age range of young people with whom CAMHS work and this, in part, defines the likely substance misuse problems the team will encounter. The spectrum includes younger children engaging in volatile substance misuse, who then progress to cannabis, stimulant and psychedelic use and later heroin use and dependence, and also potentially the use of crack cocaine. Although the main problems associated with alcohol misuse in young people relate to offending behaviour and not to help-seeking behaviour, there may be a number of young people dependent on alcohol who need appropriate detoxification and rehabilitation.

A CAMHS substance misuse team may therefore focus and advise on a number of conditions, such as attention-deficit hyperactivity disorder, conduct disorder and early formal mental illness, complicated by early or recreational substance use. If the expertise is present, the team may also provide a service for young people using crack cocaine, and for those dependent on alcohol or heroin.

Provision

As partnerships with other agencies are likely to continue to evolve, especially those with youth offending teams (YOTs) and other agencies working with young people with a high risk of substance misuse, the bare minimum that any service will provide, namely consultation, will inevitably include issues around substance misuse.

The central question seems to be how the team is able to make an accurate assessment of the degree to which substance use plays a part in the overall problem. This may be overcome if the specialist CAMHS team has a close joint working relationship with either existing adult addictions services or young people's addictions services within the voluntary or statutory sector. Alternatively, the CAMHS team could include members with both substance misuse expertise and expertise in child and adolescent mental health issues, such as adult addiction nurses who have transferred to CAMHS after taking the ENB 603 course or child psychiatrists who have become familiar with substance misuse issues through their training.

There is a feeling among adult addiction specialists that the whole gamut of interventions delivered to young substance misusers should be in the domain of child and adolescent specialists. The area that is most alien to child and adolescent psychiatrists is dealing with those young people addicted to heroin, as it opens up issues surrounding the safe prescribing of a number of opiate and non-opiate drugs. This would involve the service having the ability accurately to assess this particular client group in terms of:

- dependency
- current level of use
- mode of use

- injecting practice
- polypharmacy
- stage of motivational change.

Such assessment is necessary in order for the team to be able to deliver:

- appropriate therapeutic interventions
- appropriate prescribing interventions (stabilisation, detoxification)
- appropriate forms of detoxification (symptomatic, opiate substitute)
- interpretation of urine toxicology results
- safe dispensing and monitoring (daily collection, supervised consumption by a responsible adult).

Furthermore, in delivering these services, the team must take account of the young person's:

- education
- housing
- physical health
- mental health
- family relationships
- peer relationships
- developmental tasks
- recreation/leisure activities
- offending behaviour.

In order to deliver such a service to a group who have historically been hard to reach, the team may have to develop a more flexible approach and deliver their work in a variety of environments, such as 'one-stop shops' or on the premises of new partners. This may raise issues surrounding note keeping, confidentiality and reaching mutually agreed definitions of the young person's competence to make informed decisions about opting into treatment plans.

Treatment aims will also have to be considered: whether the goal should be abstinence from substance use, or, far more realistically, work within the broader philosophy of harm reduction. If management is shared, conflicting ideologies of service delivery may cause tensions.

Another consideration will be the provision of transitional care and the arrangements for the referral of older adolescents into appropriate adult services if they are still in need of treatment. Where community detoxification has failed or where stabilisation of the environment is required in a more intensive rehabilitation package, Tier 4 services may be required. Many child and adolescent in-patient units may exclude admission on the basis of substance misuse and many older teenagers

---

Box 24.2 Suggested reading

Abdulrahmin, D, Lavoie, D. & Hassan, S. (1999) *Commissioning Standards, Drug and Alcohol Treatment and Care*. London: Substance Misuse Advisory Service.

Crome, I. (1997) Young people and substance problems – from image to imagination (editorial). *Drugs: Education, Prevention and Policy*, **4**, 107–116.

Crome, I., Christian, J. & Green, C. (1998) Tip of the national iceberg? Profile of adolescent patients prescribed methadone in an innovative community drugs service. *Drugs: Education, Prevention and Policy*, **5**, 195–198.

Dale-Perera, A., Hamilton, C., Evans, K., *et al* (1999) *Young People and Drugs: Policy and Guidance for Drug Interventions*. Children's Legal Centre and Standing Conference on Drug Abuse.

Department of Health (1997) *The Task Force to Review Services for Drug Misusers. Report of an Independent Review of Drug Treatment Services in England*. London: Department of Health.

Department of Health (1999) *Drug Misuse and Dependence: Guidelines on Clinical Management*. London: Department of Health.

Department of Health & Social Services Inspectorate (1997) *Substance Misuse and Young People, the Social Services Response: a Social Services Inspectorate Study of Young People Looked After by Local Authorities*. London: Department of Health.

Gilvarry, E. (2000) Substance abuse in young people. *Journal of Child Psychology and Psychiatry*, **41**, 55–80.

Home Office: (1995) *Tackling Drugs Together: A Strategy for England 1995–1998*. London: HMSO.

Home Office (1998) *Tackling Drugs to Build a Better Britain: The Government's 10-year Strategy for Tackling Drug Misuse*. London: HMSO.

NHS Health Advisory Service (1996) *The Substance of Young Needs. Children's and Young People's Substance Misuse Service*. London: HMSO.

Pagliaro, A. & Pagliaro, L. (1996) *Substance Use Among Children and Adolescents: Its Nature, Extent and Effects from Conception to Adulthood*. London: John Wiley & Sons.

Parker, H., Bury, C. & Egginton, R. (1998) *New Heroin Outbreaks Amongst Young People in England and Wales*. Home Office Police Policy Directorate.

---

may also fall outside of entry criteria. Local funding arrangements may not be in place to facilitate access to the relatively few units specifically dealing with the detoxification and residential rehabilitation of young people.

Conclusion

- Substance use among young people is widespread and much discussed in the literature (Box 24.2).
- There are particular groups who are at risk of problematic substance use.

- These at-risk groups overlap with those for whom CAMHS are already being asked, along with colleagues in other children's services, to provide joined-up interventions.
- The skills already present within CAMHS – knowledge of developmental and family functioning, child-centred awareness, assessment of problems in systemic formulations and the delivery of a variety of therapeutic interventions – are essential contributions to service delivery, whether they are exercised through consultation or direct work.
- Owing to widespread geographical and inter-disciplinary differences in expertise in the field of substance misuse by children and young people, there are many models of service delivery to this group.
- Innovative partnerships and working styles may have to be developed.
- CAMHS need to contribute to strategic planning processes.
- Training needs, capacity and resources will ultimately shape the response of CAMHS to young substance users.
- The specialist CAMHS substance misuse team will need to develop smooth pathways for those who require referral to adult services or Tier 4 placements.

CHAPTER 25

Parenting risk assessment service*

Ian Partridge, Geraldine Casswell and Greg Richardson

'We may be excused for not caring much about other people's children, for there are many who care very little about their own.'
Samuel Johnson

Introduction

Multi-agency cooperation and multi-disciplinary perspectives are two prerequisites of effective child protection work (Department of Health *et al*, 1999), and this has led to structural and organisational reform in child protection investigation and assessment. The questions asked of agencies are no longer just about the establishment of the probability or certainty that a particular abusive act has taken place, but also about whether the risks of return to parental care outweigh the possible harm of statutory intervention. There is a clear requirement to demonstrate the benefit, to the child's welfare and well-being, of any intervention (Department of Health, 1991).

As understanding of the dynamics of child abuse has developed, it has become clear that risk depends on the intra-personal characteristics of parents and children and their inter-personal interactions. Mental health input into risk assessment procedures has tended to centre on the psychiatric assessment of the parenting adult and the psychological/psychiatric assessment of the child. There is, though, a role for CAMHS in looking at the parental ability to parent and the risk posed to the child's development, regardless of the absence or presence of psychiatric disturbance.

An independent multi-disciplinary team within CAMHS that assesses forensic issues within a systemic and developmental context can offer a useful contribution to the comprehensive assessment of risk and offer a valuable service to statutory agencies and the courts (Smith *et al*, 2001).

---

*This chapter is a revised version of the paper 'Assessing the risks posed by parents' previously published in *Child Psychology and Psychiatry Review* (Partridge *et al*, 2001). With permission.

The structure of the team

To command the respect of referring social services departments and the courts, such a team requires a multi-disciplinary composition of senior and experienced clinicians. It is unfortunate that, in requiring expert opinion, the courts and social services departments often undervalue the contribution of first-line workers, who are usually more familiar with the situation of, and the people involved in, these cases. Risk assessment in this field is both clinically and emotionally demanding; working within a team offers a supportive environment as well as a wider range of personal and clinical perspectives. The contribution of an agency outside social services ensures the independence of the assessment.

The philosophy of the team

- *Multi-disciplinary perspectives.* Multi-disciplinary skills and perspectives are a prerequisite of effective working in the field of child protection (Department of Health *et al*, 1999).
- *Systems theory.* To ensure that abuse is approached not only from the standpoint of the perpetrator–victim dyad but also to seek an understanding of the relational context is controversial (Bentovim *et al*, 1988; *Feminist Review*, 1988; Will, 1989). However, a wider perspective is more pertinent in both assessing risk (Elton, 1988) and informing the intervention/non-intervention debate.
- *Developmental context.* A child's welfare is dependent on the parent's or carer's ability to adapt to the child's development. Attachment theory (Bowlby, 1982; Rutter, 1981) provides a structure to explore the childhood experiences of parents and how they contribute to, or interfere with, the care of their children (Crittenden & Ainsworth, 1989; George, 1996).
- *Forensic context.* The only real indicator of risk is a previous history of abusive behaviour. This fact requires the questioning of the potential for change within developmentally acceptable time-scales and the generation of strategies for the management of risk within a system either with or without additional support and monitoring. A multi-factorial model of understanding risk is the most helpful (Finkelhor, 1986).

Managing referrals

All referrals to a risk assessment service are necessarily complex and arise from concerns about the protection of children. It is usual that court cases are proceeding or pending. Invariably, the work will be requested in the context of ongoing child protection case conferences; it is therefore probable that the legal department of the local authority will be closely involved with the case.

Initial contact with the service will often be by telephone, from an involved professional. This allows preliminary discussion of the appropriateness of the referral as well as discussion of time-scales for the assessment and report. This must be followed by a more detailed written referral, accompanied by relevant documentation. Where the referral takes place in the context of court proceedings, there should be a letter of instruction from the appropriate legal agencies, with a clear articulation of the questions the team is being asked to address (see Chapter 10).

Following referral, a professional meeting should be arranged at which members of the risk assessment team meet all the professionals and carers involved with the care of the children in the subject family. This meeting has three main objectives:

- to share background information on the case and to discuss the value of a risk assessment in the context of the current situation and previous assessments by other agencies and teams
- to clarify (and to agree and document) the specific questions the risk assessment team is being asked to address, and those issues the team will not be addressing (the team must never act beyond its competence)
- to agree the input of all agencies into the risk assessment, to ensure a comprehensive, integrated multi-agency assessment.

In addition, time-scales for both assessment and presentation of the report will need to be negotiated. A member of the team should be nominated to speak in court if necessary. The communication network and points of contact should be established. The dates of the assessment sessions should be given to the responsible social worker and appointment letters sent to the appropriate family members.

This meeting is most appropriately chaired by a member of the risk assessment team and will be recorded. A further professionals' meeting will be arranged for feedback of the assessment. There will be occasions when the family and, in particularly contentious cases, their legal representatives will be present at this meeting.

The assessment process

The assessment (Box 25.1) will be geared to the concerns of the referring agency, and also to the nature of the case referred. However, the team should have a clear focus for its work, which is the assessment of the risk posed by the parents or carers or other adults involved, or potentially involved, with the children. The team offers only a contribution to the risk assessment process – its assessment must be taken in conjunction

Box 25.1 Framework of assessment

- The relevance of the psychological and psychiatric state of the child's parents, their partners and other relevant family members, to their parenting skills.
- The factors relevant to parenting in the relationship between the parents (or parent and partner).
- The availability of supportive factors in the parents' environment.
- The parents' willingness to avail themselves of support in parenting.

with other assessments offered by other agencies and professionals.

The areas subject to assessment are considered in relation to risks posed to the child's safety and welfare (Box 25.2). Often there have already been incidents of abuse and neglect; in other cases there is, at the very least, a strong concern that the child's developmental welfare is or will be impaired as a result of the parenting received.

To address the questions of concern, a series of four or five assessment sessions or a whole-day assessment (Wheeler *et al*, 1998) provide the time to work with the parents as a couple, as well as the opportunity to engage in individually focused assessment. To provide gender balance, it may be helpful for two therapists to undertake the assessment, with live supervision provided by the other team members. The family should receive feedback and receive a copy of the assessment report. The report should be sent to the referrer for distribution to all relevant agencies.

Box 25.2 Factors in assessing risk

- The abusing parent's understanding of the abuse or neglect, or potential abuse or neglect.
- The non-abusing parent's understanding of the abuse or neglect, or potential abuse or neglect.
- The parents' understanding of the parental task, related to an understanding of the child's developmental needs.
- The ability and resources to change in order to become a 'good enough' parent.
- The additional support or treatment required for the parents to change, and their willingness to use such support.

CHAPTER 26

Forensic services

Sue Bailey

'only connect'
E. M. Forster

Introduction

Young people at the interface of the criminal justice system and mental health services face social exclusion, alienation and stigmatisation (Bailey, 1999). The definition of this group varies across and within agencies; their needs are diverse and require a range of mental health services that can be effective only if integrated with the services of other agencies.

Young people account for an estimated 7 million crimes a year. The psychosocial and biological factors placing young people at risk of both offending and mental health problems are well established (Junger-Tas, 1994; Kazdin, 1995; Rutter & Smith, 1995; Shepherd & Farrington, 1996; Rutter et al, 1998; Rutter, 1999).

Definitions

Forensic mental health has been defined as an area of specialisation that involves the assessment and treatment of those who are both mentally disordered and whose behaviour has led or could lead to offending (Mullen, 2000). Defining forensic psychiatry in terms of the assessment and treatment of the mentally abnormal offender delineates an area of concern that could engulf much of mental health. Offending behaviour is common in the whole community and, as Mullen notes, among adolescents it approaches the universal, with 50% of all known offenders being under the age of 21. Criminal convictions are spread widely through society and even more widely among people with mental disorders. In practice, patients often gravitate to adult forensic services when the nature of their offending or the anxiety and apprehension created by their behaviour is such as to overwhelm the tolerance or confidence of professionals in the general mental health services. In part, these cases are also driven by the emerging culture of blame, in which professionals fear being held responsible for failing to protect their fellow citizens from the violent behaviour of those who have been in their care. Mullen (2000) stresses that mental health expertise should address the mental health component of social problems, and highlights the importance of rigorous risk assessments and management.

There is an association between substance misuse, mental disorder and offending. Nowhere is this more important than in the field of adolescent forensic psychiatry.

Background

In England and Wales during the past 20 years there have been major changes in legislation that were meant to bring about an improvement in services to children. The Children Act 1989 reformed the law, and brought public and private law under one statutory system. Section 37 of the Crime and Disorder Act 1998 lays the statutory duty on services, including health, education, the police, probation and local authority social services, to prevent crime through effective inter-agency practice and appropriate forms of intervention.

Surveys of young people at different points in the criminal justice system both in the UK and in the USA show high rates of psychiatric disorder, particularly among persistent offenders (Dolan *et al*, 1999; Kazdin, 2000; Lader *et al*, 2000). Despite some positive policy moves in the UK (Harding, 1999), a large number still end up remanded or sentenced to custody, and this is illustrated by the rising number of young people and children who now find themselves in the new secure state provision. This includes over 2500 young people incarcerated, at any one time, in local authority secure childrens' homes, young offender institutions, secure psychiatric units and secure training centres.

When young people become involved in the detention justice system, the focus on their offending behaviour tends to take precedence over developmental and mental health issues. The young offender with a mental health problem tends to fall in the gap between the organisational boundaries of different agencies, such as social services, youth offending teams, educational provision and CAMHS. Of particular concern to probation services are those over 16 years of age, some of whom do not have access to a general practitioner. The absence of a holistic approach is starkly apparent; there is no provision for identified key workers, as set out with the Care Programme Approach, to maintain continuity of care for the young person.

The 1997 *Thematic Review of Young Prisoners* (HM Inspectorate of Prisons, 1997) found that, between the ages of 16 and 24, mental and emotional difficulties are major problems for young people in prison. Over 50% of remanded young males and over 30% of sentenced young males have a diagnosable mental disorder. At every level of intervention, from the entry point of prison reception, the excessive delay in transferring the assessed patient from the prison to the National Health Service (NHS), to the fragmented arrangements for care after release, the report chronicles a range of failings. The report argues that these failings can be addressed only by the NHS taking over a responsibility for the health care of young people in custody, so that there is more consistency with provision offered in the community. This becomes more important when the rise in the suicide rate for young men over recent years is considered. In 1996, 547 men between the ages of 15 and 24 took their own lives in the UK. The multi-disciplinary youth offending teams established by the Crime and Disorder Act have aided the coordination and cooperation for offenders under 18 years. However, such cooperation can be effective only if there are resources within CAMHS and professionals trained and willing to do the job.

Problem profiles

The assessment of a young person whose mental health is called into question is the responsibility of the locality CAMHS. It should be the first port of call for those dealing with young offenders, such as social workers or youth offending teams. Such work will require resourcing and prioritising. Scott (1998) stresses the need for CAMHS to offer an integrated assessment with other agencies. The aim is to work with young children with antisocial behaviour in a family context using parent management training strategies, combined with individual interventions for the young person, which take into account subtyping of conduct disorder based on age of onset.

The long-term follow-up studies of young people in secure care appear to demonstrate five routes into offending (Bullock & Millam 1998):

- young people in long-term care
- young people requiring prolonged special education
- young people whose behaviour suddenly deteriorated in adolescence
- one-off grave offenders
- serious and persistent offenders.

Broad and overlapping sets of problems associated with offending have been identified and will need to be addressed concurrently. Rutter *et al* (1998) stress the heterogeneity of antisocial behaviour, in terms of the pervasiveness, persistence, severity and patterns of such behaviour. Comorbid factors with youth offending include:

- attention-deficit hyperactivity disorders (Scott, 1998)
- the early onset of antisocial behaviour, which includes aggressive, violent, disruptive behaviour, coercive sexual activity, arson and fluctuations in mood state and levels of social interaction
- sexual offences
- juvenile homicide
- drug use and misuse, which have increased rapidly over the past ten years
- repetitive high-risk behaviours, such as female adolescents presenting with serious suicide attempts and self-mutilation interspersed with externalising destructive behaviours – such young people raise grave anxieties within existing service provision, but even here violent behaviour in girls is underestimated, partly owing to the non-specific and insensitive diagnostic criteria for conduct disorders in girls (Jasper *et al*, 1998)
- sexual and physical abuse in the previous lives of offending boys who also go on to self-harm
- mental illness, which may have a lead-in period of one to seven years to early-onset psychosis, during which time there is a marked variation in the degree of non-psychotic behaviour and disturbance (the importance of the accurate assessment of young offenders who show multiple high-risk episodes associated with a fluctuating mental state needs to be more fully recognised)
- learning disability.

Situations of particular vulnerability and risk are homelessness and penal remand detention. Interconnections between homelessness, mental disorders, substance misuse and offending are complex and remain poorly understood.

The risk in adult life for both girls and boys is the development of personality disorder. The full range of psychological therapies should be available to those vulnerable adolescents, particularly those leaving care and at risk of custody (Royal College of Psychiatrists, 1999*a*). Multi-systemic therapy, with family- and community-based interventions, can be effective in terms of improved clinical outcomes and cost savings (Hengeller, 1999).

Addressing the problem

Young offenders require:

- a strategic approach to commissioning and delivering services for them (this approach must develop effective and predictable services that meet their current and future needs, build upon established concepts of service, and ensure that workforce planning issues are addressed and met by longer-term training)

- a better understanding of young offenders' needs across all involved agencies, which must also develop local inter-agency strategies, such as flexible working in court diversion schemes with innovative partnerships with the voluntary sector (Maziade *et al*, 1997)
- access to primary health care
- speedy access to CAMHS, as their needs are unlikely to be met by adult mental health services
- an overcoming of the reluctance to accept them into services, despite the fear of stigmatising the young people
- speedy access to drug and alcohol education and treatment centres (intensive forms of intervention for drug users with complex care needs would involve specialist residential services and mental health teams closely linked to CAMHS and forensic services)
- speedy access to HIV testing
- improved inter-agency training of non-health professionals in identifying the indicators of mental vulnerability in young people, thus strengthening the communications with professionals in the mental health services
- recognition that adolescents with learning disability will have a slower pace of developing coping strategies and changing, which must always be balanced against their risk to others
- awareness by all agencies of gaps in the capacity of existing services
- the establishment, on a regional basis, of adolescent forensic mental health teams (Box 26.1).

There is also a need for social regimes that help to promote the health of young people in prison. A joint Prison Service/NHS working group recommended a partnership to improve the health care provided

---

Box 26.1 Purposes and aims of an adolescent forensic mental health team

- Improved outreach services.
- The extension of court psychiatric schemes and pre-court diversion to youth courts.
- The development of programmes for young people before they reach the courts and custody, including adolescent in-patient services and access to secure forensic facilities.
- Post-custodial rehabilitation and support for young offenders.
- A shared approach to risk assessment and management, together with agreed protocols for better information exchange, between the health service and criminal justice agencies.
- An awareness of professional practice and service developments and research.

to prisoners and recognised the importance of a healthy prison regime (HM Prison Service, 1999). Girls and young people from ethnic minorities are recognised to be particularly vulnerable to aversive prison regimes. However, at present, there are no specialised facilities available for young girls in prison: 16- and 17-year-olds still find themselves in adult female prisons.

There is a drive for the specialist assessment, management and treatment of adolescents who display the criminal behaviours of interpersonal violence, arson and sexual offences. The focus should be on developmental issues, in contrast to the past tendency to apply adult treatment models to young people (Vizard & Usiskin, 1999).

Young people should be referred to a specialist forensic service only if they have been assessed locally to require such resources. Local multi-agency interventions must take priority.

Solutions

Ways to develop services have been described from assessments of need, commissioning exercises and clinical experience (Kurtz *et al*, 1997; Bailey & Farnworth, 1998; Audit Commission, 1999; Knapp & Henderson, 1999).

A review of the adolescent forensic service at Salford's Prestwick hospital (NHS Health Advisory Service *et al*, 1994) concluded that the greatest immediate need was for an increase in secure NHS-funded provision for:

- mentally disordered offenders
- sex offenders and abusers
- severely suicidal and self-harming adolescents
- very severely mentally ill adolescents
- adolescents who need to begin psychiatric rehabilitation in secure circumstances
- brain-injured adolescents and those with severe organic disorders.

Some of these services are being developed in the independent sector.

A framework for services

A strategic framework for youth offender mental health services would be a four-tier model in which local generic and regional specialist services allow for the multi-dimensional problems encountered by these young people to be tackled by local CAMHS in conjunction with other agencies. The four tiers would comprise:

- *Local CAMHS provision for young offenders*, while ensuring resources for the rest of the locality CAMHS are not depleted by this work.

- *Local CAMHS augmented* by advice and training offered by a peripatetic outreach team that is based in and works from specialised centres of expertise in forensic child and adolescent mental health. These patients are highly mobile, as their families frequently move from one local authority to another and their residential placements often change. Funding and services must follow the child, and not be obstructed by agency and geographical boundaries, to ensure continuity of care.
- *Peripatetic specialised forensic services* in which the young people are seen directly by members of an outreach service from a specialised centre of expertise, sharing responsibility with the locality CAMHS.
- *Tier 4 centres of specialist forensic expertise*, which deliver services directly to patients and their families. This may involve open units, high-dependency units and intensive assessment and care units, with security between medium and high, and considerable emphasis being placed on staff training and the dissemination of expertise.

Such a strategic framework is ambitious and requires:

- staff wanting to work in this area
- comprehensive training systems
- evidence-based interventions
- a national adolescent forensic mental health research and development network, which has now been established, to ensure that what is learnt from research is promptly put into practice.

Since April 2000, there has been central commissioning (by the National Specialist Commissioning Advisory Group) for developed and developing adolescent forensic secure psychiatric in-patient units in England, with a strengthening of an adolescent forensic practitioner network

Conclusion

The government strategy for modernising mental health services (Department of Health, 1998a) put forward, for the first time, a health strategy with risk assessment and public protection as top priorities. Child and adolescent mental health professionals have traditionally been involved at the interface between the law and the welfare of children, but historically this has often been via the need for their professional opinion on children in the child care system rather than in forensic matters. CAMHS are important in helping professionals in other agencies to recognise developmental and interactional influences on offending behaviour.

CHAPTER 27

Neuropsychology and neuropsychiatry services

Helen Prescott and Ian Partridge

'Good practice requires not simply the collection of test data and observation, but the interpretation of this data in the context of age, developmental stage, injury/insult severity and psychosocial context.'
Anderson *et al* (2001)

Introduction

Neurological disorders account for around one-third of all cases of paediatric illness (Kennedy, 1998). Paediatric neurology is one of the larger specialities and provides a service for children affected by many and diverse disorders. Paediatric neuropsychological support has been recognised as deficient. In its 'Blue Book' (Kennedy, 1998) submission, the British Paediatric Neurology Association assigned it a high priority for remedial action, and indicated that such support is an essential component of a paediatric neurology service.

Children with neuropsychological problems require specialist provision. This area has been under-recognised in the development of CAMHS and services have been provided in an ad hoc fashion, usually developing out of research centres and operating on a supra-regional level. Owing to lack of service provision, clinicians working with adults have had children referred to them. Such referrals have often led to the application of adult models of neuropsychology to children, sometimes without due consideration of the unique and complex issues related to childhood and adolescence.

Establishing a service

In the establishment of a neuropsychological service, the following conceptual points require consideration:

- *How adult neuropsychology differs from child neuropsychology –* including consideration of the concepts of development and maturation. Concepts of localisation are more limited in children and therefore it is more difficult to establish clear brain–behaviour relationships. Damage sustained by children tends to be more diffuse, less focal and tends to produce more generalised cognitive effects.

- *Age effects*. The age and developmental status of the child at time of injury or insult will influence short- and long-term outcome. Age at assessment will also reveal different effects of injury or insult, as there will be latent or sleeper effects.
- *Brain–behaviour models* – structural development of the central nervous system and its correlation with specific behaviours.

Over recent years there has been both a wider application of neuropsychological models in clinical practice and an increase in understanding of children's neurodevelopment (Middleton, 2000). By implication, there is a need for effective and coordinated child neuropsychological services.

There needs to be an effective clinical response to the following:

- traumatic brain injury
- neurodegenerative diseases
- brain tumours
- epilepsy
- acute viral illnesses (e.g. encephalitis, meningitis)
- developmental disorders
- childhood strokes
- specific learning difficulties
- non-specific disorders (e.g. migraine)
- non-organic presentations
- neuromuscular diseases
- neurological aspects of multi-system disease.

A child neuropsychological service requires a core multi-disciplinary team working in a clear inter-disciplinary and inter-agency fashion. This team should consist of:

- a clinical psychologist
- a psychiatrist
- a specialist liaison nurse or health visitor
- a social worker.

There should be established clear networks and working links with:

- occupational therapists
- physiotherapists
- speech and language therapists
- paediatric neurologists
- paediatric oncologists
- endocrinologists
- haematologists

- radiologists
- education staff.

In establishing neuropsychological/neuropsychiatric provision, there will be a need to manage the available resources and to maintain a clear overview of the demands upon the service and its development. The process of allocation should be based upon a clear identification of the functions of the various team members. This area of provision is part of a larger and wider service and, as such, emphasis must be placed upon the marrying up of services in a clear and integrated fashion. Clear networks of communication will be essential for the service to be relevant to the needs of children and families.

There should be an operational policy regarding neuropsychological provision.

Operation

Most referrals to a neuropsychological service come from the medical services. CAMHS has a clear role to inform the whole intervention with the child and family. For CAMHS to operate an effective neuropsychological service, consideration must be given to the following areas.

Assessment

The assessment will encompass specific neuropsychological issues, as well as the family and social context. Assessment may be triggered by:

- concerns about developmental progress
- the need to investigate neurodevelopmental status
- concern about general or specific cognitive abilities
- the need to establish a baseline, to enable monitoring of change
- the need to investigate the consequences of a specific event
- hypothesis testing.

The assessment will involve informal and formal investigation and will work from a multi-factorial, interactional model, with full evaluation of both biological factors and neurodevelopmental experience.

Assessment is therefore informed by a detailed history that includes:

- prenatal and birth history
- full developmental history
- attachment and social history
- systemic factors
- detailed psychometric assessment, including serial testing
- assessment of family resources, for example with regard to the impact of surgical interventions and the operation of treatment regimes (including medication)

- assessment of the child's resources and coping strategies with regard to both the presenting problem and the nature of the intervention.

Interventions

- *Clarification of the problem.* It is important to recognise that the assessment offered is central to informing all interventions and in particular the nature and scope of the medical interventions. The assessment has the function of making the problems more explicit and clearly defined, and this will help external agencies, such as schools, that have day-to-day dealings with the child and family.
- *Advice and information.* This will be important for the child, the family and external agencies, including statutory and voluntary agencies.
- *Strategies for the individual.* These strategies will aim to enable children to attain or recover physical, psychological and social function to the greatest degree possible.
- *Strategies for the family.* These strategies will help the children and their families to make a healthy adaptation to their circumstances.
- *Inter-agency networking.* The CAMHS should liaise with education services and other community-based health services in order that appropriate services can be planned as close to the child's home as possible.

Conclusion

Child clinical neuropsychology is a growing, but still very small, field of applied psychology in the UK. Although much can be transferred from the field of adult neuropsychology, there are many important differences between working with children and with adults. The most important of these differences is the rapidly changing course of neurological development throughout childhood, along with equally rapidly changing environmental demands. Knowledge of normal development, of specific issues relating to children and of the networks of which they are part is therefore essential. There is also potential for applying clinical neuropsychological models where treatments have neuropsychological effects, and to specific learning difficulties in children. A multi-disciplinary neuropsychological child mental health service has an essential role in enhancing the range and quality of health care provided by a paediatric neurosciences service.

Glossary

Centre for Evidence Based Child Health
Aims to help practitioners gain skills in integrating evidence from research into the clinical practice of child health (http://www. gosh.nhs.uk/ich/html/academicunits/paed_epid/cebch/about.html).

Centre for Evidence Based Mental Health
Provides access to the journal *Evidence-Based Mental Health* and a 'tool kit' of useful resources for evidence-based practice (http:// cebmh.warne.ox.ac.uk/cebmh).

Conventional reviews
Reviews of the scientific literature that do not necessarily contain all the relevant available studies and often contain an unknown amount of subjective opinion. Systematic reviews (q.v.) are preferable.

Evidence-based medicine (EBM)
Defined by Sackett *et al* (1997) as 'the conscientious, explicit and judicious use of, current best evidence, in making decisions about the care of individual patients'. As such conscientious, explicit and judicious use of current best evidence is the responsibility of all health care professionals, the preferred term used in this volume is evidence-based practice (EBP).

Evidence-based practice (EBP)
see evidence-based medicine (EBM).

FOCUS
A Royal College of Psychiatrists' project to promote effective practice in CAMHS (http://www.rcpsych.ac.uk/cru/focus). It can be joined without charge by any member of a CAMHS. FOCUS produces a news-letter and a free guide to useful websites and online journals for CAMHS professionals. (Contact: Catherine Ayres at FOCUS, Royal College of Psychiatrists' Research Unit, 6th floor, 83 Victoria Street, London SW1H 0HW. Tel: 020 7227 0822. Email: catherine.ayres@virgin.net.)

Host organisation

Any organisation that is responsible for the management of CAMHS provision. The term may therefore describe a mental health trust, a primary care trust, an acute trust, a social care trust, or any similar organisation with this responsibility.

Medical responsibility

A complex concept, which has been used to engender considerable anxiety in doctors by making them feel responsible for all that happens to people involved in services to which they have professional commitment. Interestingly, two recent publications from the General Medical Council, *Management in Health Care: The Role of Doctors* (1999) and *Good Medical Practice* (2001), make no reference to medical responsibility. Similarly, the Royal College of Psychiatrists does not list medical responsibility in its document on good practice (Royal College of Psychiatrists, 2000). All three documents call attention to a doctor's responsibilities when working in multi-disciplinary teams. If medical responsibility is viewed as performing the duties of a doctor, effective multi-disciplinary working is assured. The practice of each professional in CAMHS is his/her responsibility, for which he/she will receive professional supervision and support.

Mental disorder

Implies the existence of a clinically recognisable set of symptoms or behaviours associated in most cases with distress and with interference with personal functions (NHS Health Advisory Service, 1995*a*).

Mental health problems

Can arise from a young person's difficulties in coping with life, developmental difficulty, the impact of sensory handicap or educational difficulty or from social difficulties (NHS Health Advisory Service, 1995*a*).

Meta-analysis

Involves the mathematical synthesis of the results of a number of randomised controlled trials that have addressed the same question in the same way, with added weight being given to the bigger studies.

NICE

National Institute of Clinical Excellence (http://www.nice.org.uk).

Portage worker

A community-based professional who works with pre-school children with learning difficulties and disabilities and their carers in their homes. The purpose of the work is to stimulate the child's development through the carer–child relationship.

Responsible medical officer

A term defined in the Mental Health Act 1983. It is sometimes more widely used, but its use in this handbook will be confined to that definition.

Special educational needs coordinator

A member of staff in a school who takes responsibility for coordinating multi-agency responses to pupils within the school who have special needs.

Systematic reviews

Reviews of the scientific literature in which the reviewer uses rigorous, explicit, defined methods to find all the primary studies in the literature (usually randomised controlled trials). Those with reliable, valid results are then summarised. Poor-quality studies are discarded. The Cochrane Collaboration is a major source of these high-quality systematic reviews and makes abstracts of these available on the Internet (http://www.update-software.com/cochrane).

References

Abbot, S., Johnson, L., Henwood, M., *et al* (1998) *A Continuing Challenge: Evaluation of the Implementation of Continuing Care Guidance: Final Report.* Leeds: Community Care Division of the Nuffield Institute for Health, University of Leeds.

Abdulrahmin, D., Lavoie, D. & Hassan, S. (1999) *Commissioning Standards, Drug and Alcohol Treatment and Care.* London: Substance Misuse Advisory Service.

Achenbach, T. (1991) *Integrative Guide for the 1991 CBCL/4–18, YSR, and TRF Profiles.* Burlington, VT: University of Vermont Department of Psychiatry.

Adcock, M. & White, R. (1998) *Significant Harm.* Croydon: Significant Publications.

American Association on Mental Retardation (1992) *Mental Retardation: Definition, Classifications and Systems of Support* (9th revision). Washington, DC: AAMR.

Anderson, V., Northam, E., Hendry, J., *et al* (2001) *Developmental Neuropsychology: A Clinical Approach.* Hove: Psychology Press.

Andrews, J. A. & Lewinsohn, P. M. (1992) Suicidal attempts among older adolescents: prevalence and co-occurrence with psychiatric disorders. *Journal of the American Academy of Child and Adolescent Psychiatry*, **31**, 655–662.

Anonymous (1997) Emergency admissions: an open letter. *Young Minds*, **31**, 6–8.

Appeal Cases (1986) Gillick *v.* West Midlands and Wisbech Area Health Authority. Law Report AC 112.

Asperger, H. (1944) Die autistischen psychopathen im kindesalter. *Archiv für Psychiatrie und Nervenkrankheiten*, **117**, 76–136.

Audit Commission (1992) *Getting in on the Act. Provision for Pupils with Special Educational Needs: The National Picture.* London: HMSO.

—— (1999) *Children in Mind.* London: Audit Commission Publications.

Bailey, S. (1999) The interface between mental health, criminal justice and forensic mental health services for children and adolescents. *Current Opinion in Psychiatry*, **12**, 425–428.

—— & Farnworth, P. (1998) Forensic mental health services. *Young Minds Magazine*, **34**, 12–13.

Bakwin, H. (1957) Suicide in children and adolescents. *Journal of Paediatrics*, **50**, 749–769.

Balk, D. E. (1990) The self concept of bereaved adolescents: sibling death and its aftermath. *Journal of Adolescent Research*, **5**, 112–132.

Bandura, A., Adams, N. E., Hardy, A .B., *et al* (1980) Tests of the generality of the self-efficacy theory. *Cognitive Therapy and Research*, **4**, 39–66.

Barkley, R. A. (1990) *Attention Deficit Hyperactivity Disorder: A Handbook for Diagnosis and Treatment.* New York: Guilford Press.

Baron-Cohen, S., Allen, J. & Gillberg, C. (1992) Can autism be detected at 18 months? The needle, the haystack and the CHAT. *British Journal of Psychiatry*, **161**, 839–843.

Bartlet, L. B. (1996) School pressures and child mental health in Afro-Asian countries. *Psychiatric Bulletin*, **20**, 301–303.

Baulkwill, J. & Wood, C. (1994) Group work with bereaved children. *European Journal of Palliative Care*, **1**, 113–115.

Beelman, A., Pfingset, U. & Losel, F. (1994) Effects of training social competence in children: a meta-analysis of recent evaluation studies. *Journal of Clinical Child Psychology*, **23**, 260–271.

Bentovim, A., Elton, A., Hildebrand, J., *et al* (1988) *Child Sexual Abuse Within the Family: Assessment and Treatment*. London: Wright.

Bhui, K. & Moran, T. (1995) Who uses a residential child psychiatry unit? *ACCP Review and Newsletter*, **17**, 309–312.

Bickman, L., Foster, E. M. & Lambert, E. W. (1996) Who gets hospitalised in a continuum of care? *Journal of the American Academy of Child and Adolescent Psychiatry*, **35**, 74–80.

Bifulco, A. T., Brown, G. W. & Harris, T. O. (1987) Childhood loss of a parent, lack of parental care and adult depression: a replication. *Journal of Affective Disorders*, **12**, 115–128.

Bingley, L., Leonard, J., Hensman, S., *et al* (1980) The comprehensive management of children on a paediatric ward – a family approach. *Archives of Disease in Childhood*, **55**, 555–561.

Bishop, D. (1989) *Test for Reception of Grammar (TROG)*. Manchester: University of Manchester.

Black, D. (1996) Roles, responsibilities and work of a child and adolescent psychiatrist. In *Child and Adolescent Psychiatry. A New Century* (Occasional Paper OP33) (eds J. Harris-Hendricks & M. Black), pp. 17–24. London: Royal College of Psychiatrists.

— , McFadyen, A. & Broster, G. (1990) Development of a psychiatric liaison service. *Archives of Disease in Childhood*, **65**, 1373–1375.

— , Harris-Hendricks, J. & Wolkind, S. (eds) (1998) *Child Psychiatry and the Law* (3rd edn). London: Gaskell.

— , Wright, B., Williams, C., *et al* (1999) Paediatric liaison service. *Psychiatric Bulletin*, **23**, 528–530.

Blackwell, B. & Currah, J. (1973) The psychopharmacology of nocturnal enuresis. In *Bladder Control and Enuresis* (eds I. Kolvin, R. C. MacKeith & S. R. Meadow), pp. 231–257. London: Heinemann.

Bowlby, J. (1980) *Attachment, Vol. III. Loss, Sadness and Depression*. London: Hogarth Press.

— (1982) *Attachment, Vol. I. Attachment and Loss*. London: Hogarth Press.

Bramble, D. (1998) Attention deficit hyperactivity disorder. Child psychiatrists should help parents with difficult children, not blame them. *BMJ*, **317**, 1250–1251.

British Medical Association (2001) *Report of the Consent Working Party: Incorporating Consent Tool Kit*. London: BMA.

British Psychological Society (1993) *Purchasing Clinical Psychology Services: Services for Children, Young People and their Families*. Leicester: British Psychological Society.

— (2000) *Managing Litigation Arising in Clinical Work with Children and Families*. Leicester: BPS.

— (2001) *SIG Position Paper: Practice Guidance on Consent for Clinical Psychologists Working with Children and Young People*. Leicester: BPS.

Brophy, J. (2001) *Child Psychiatry and Child Protection Litigation*. London: Gaskell.

— , Wale, C. J. & Bates, P. (1999) *Myths and Practices: A National Survey of the Use of Experts in Child Care Proceedings*. London: British Agencies for Adoption and Fostering.

Brown, A. & Cooper, A. F. (1987) The impact of a liaison psychiatry service on patterns of referral in a general hospital. *British Journal of Psychiatry*, **150**, 83–87.

Brown, J. (1994) *The Hybrid Worker – Lessons Based Upon a Study of Employers Involved with Two Pioneer Joint Qualifying Training Courses*. London: Central Council for Education and Training in Social Work

Brown, M. (1996) Day patient treatment. In *Child Psychiatric Units: At the Crossroads* (eds R. Chesson & D. Chisholm), pp. 45–52. London: Jessica Kingsley.

Bullock, R. & Millam, S. (1998) *Secure Treatment Outcomes: The Care Careers of Very Difficult Adolescents*. Dartington: Ashgate.

Bury, T. & Mead, J. (1998) *Evidence-Based Healthcare: A Practical Guide for Therapists*. London: Heinemann.

Butler-Sloss, E. (1987) *Report of the Inquiry into Child Abuse in Cleveland 1987*. London: HMSO.

Byford, S., Harrington, R., Torgerson, D., *et al* (1999) Cost-effectiveness analysis of a home-based social work intervention for children and adolescents who have deliberately poisoned themselves. Results of a randomised controlled trial. *British Journal of Psychiatry*, **174**, 56–62.

Cantwell, D. P. & Baker, L. (1992) Association between attention deficit hyperactivity disorder and learning disorders. In *Attention Deficit Disorder Comes of Age: Towards the Twenty-First Century* (eds S. E. Shaywitz & B. A. Shaywitz), pp. 145–164. Austin, TX: Pro-Ed.

Carson, D. (1990) *Risk Taking in Mental Disorder: Analyses, Policies and Practical Strategies*. Chichester: SLE Publications.

Chambers, R. (1994*a*) Participatory rural appraisal: challenges, potentials and paradigm. *World Development*, **22**(10).

— (1994*b*) The origins and practice of participatory rural appraisal. *World Development*, **22**(7).

— (1998) *Clinical Effectiveness Made Easy. First Thoughts on Clinical Governance*. Oxford: Radcliffe Medical Press.

Citizens Commission on Human Rights (1995) *Psychiatry: Education's Ruin*. London: CCHR International.

Cohen, D. & Volkmar, F. (1997) *Handbook of Autism and Pervasive Developmental Disorders*. New York: Wiley.

Corbett, J. A. (1985) Mental retardation: psychiatric aspects. In *Child and Adolescent Psychiatry* (eds M. Rutter & L. Hersov), pp. 661–678. Oxford: Blackwell Scientific.

Cornwall, A. & Jewkes, R. (1995) What is participatory research? *Social Science and Medicine*, **41** (12).

Cottrell, D. & Worrall, A. (1995) Liaison child and adolescent psychiatry. *Advances in Psychiatric Treatment*, **1**, 78–85.

—, Hill, P., Walk, D., *et al* (1988) Factors influencing non-attendance at child psychiatry out-patient appointments. *British Journal of Psychiatry*, **152**, 201–204.

Cox, A. (1994) Diagnostic appraisal. In *Child and Adolescent Psychiatry: Modern Approaches* (eds M. Rutter, E. Taylor & L. Hersov), pp. 22–33. Oxford: Blackwell Scientific.

Creed, F., Mbaya, P., Lancashire, S., *et al* (1997) Cost effectiveness of day and inpatient psychiatric treatment: results of a randomised controlled trial. *BMJ*, **314**, 1381–1385.

Critten, P. (1993) *Investing in People: Towards Corporate Capability*. Oxford: Butterworth.

Crittenden, P. & Ainsworth, M. D. S. (1989) Child maltreatment and attachment theory. In *Handbook of Child Maltreatment: Clinical and Theoretical Perspectives*. New York: Cambridge University Press.

Cullen, D. (1992) *Child Care Law. A Summary of the Law in England and Wales*. London: British Agencies for Adoption and Fostering.

Cunningham, C. E., Bremner, R. & Boyle, M. (1995) Large group community based parenting programs for families of preschoolers at risk for disruptive behaviour disorders: utilization, cost effectiveness and outcome. *Journal of Child Psychology and Psychiatry*, **36**, 1141–1159.

Davies, G. & Ames, S. (1998) Adolescents referred following overdose. *Psychiatric Bulletin*, **22**, 359–361.

Davison, I. (1996) Innovation and efficacy: the challenges of a new children's day resource. *Child Psychology and Psychiatry Review*, **1**, 26–30.

De Shazer, S. (1985) *Keys to Solutions in Brief Therapy*. New York: Norton.

— (1988) *Clues: Investigating Solutions in Brief Therapy*. New York: Norton.

De Silva, P., Dodds, P., Rainey, J., *et al* (1995) Management and the multidisciplinary team. In *Management for Psychiatrists* (2nd edn) (eds D. Bhugra & A. Burns), pp. 121–138. London: Gaskell.

Department for Education and Skills (2001*a*) *Promoting Children's Mental Health Within Early Years and School Settings.* Nottingham: DfEE Publications.

— (2001*b*) *Special Educational Needs Code of Practice.* Nottingham: DfES Publications.

Department of Health (1988) *Working Together: A Guide to Arrangements for the Protection of Children from Abuse.* London: HMSO.

— (1990) *Joint Health and Social Services Council: The Care Programme Approach for People with a Mental Illness Referred to Specialist Psychiatric Services.* London: Department of Health.

— (1991) *Introduction to the Children Act 1989.* London: HMSO.

— (1993) *Working Together for Better Health.* London: Department of Health.

— (1997*a*) *The New NHS: Modern, Dependable.* London: Stationery Office.

— (1997*b*) *The Task Force to Review Services for Drug Misusers. Report of an Independent Review of Drug Treatment Services in England.* London: Department of Health.

— (1998*a*) *Modernising Mental Health Services.* London: Department of Health.

— (1998*b*) *Our Healthier Nation: A Contract for Health.* London: Stationery Office.

— (1998*c*) *A First Class Service: Quality in the New NHS.* London: Stationery Office.

— (1999*a*) *NHS Modernisation Fund and Mental Health Grant for Child and Adolescent Mental Health Services 1999/2002* (Health Service Circular 1999/126; Local Authority Circular (99), 22). London: Department of Health.

— (1999*b*) *Quality Protects Programme: Transforming Childrens' Services.* London: Department of Health.

— (2000*a*) *The Government's Response to the Health Select Committee's Report into Mental Health Services.* London: Stationery Office.

— (2000*b*) *The NHS Plan.* London: Department of Health.

— (2000*c*) *Framework for the Assessment of Children in Need and Their Families.* London: Stationery Office.

— (2001*a*) *Consent – What You Have a Right to Expect: A Guide for Children and Young People.* London: Department of Health.

— (2001*b*) *Seeking Consent: Working With Children.* London: Department of Health.

— (2001*c*) *Valuing People: A New Strategy for Learning Disability for the 21st Century.* London: Stationery Office.

— (2001*d*) *The Journey to Recovery – The Government's Vision for Mental Health Care.* London: Department of Health.

— (2001*e*) *Reference Guide to Consent for Examination or Treatment.* London: Department of Health.

— (2001*f*) *Assuring the Quality of Medical Practice. Implementing Supporting Doctors Protecting Patients.* London: Department of Health.

— (2002*a*) *National Suicide Prevention Strategy for England: Consultation Document.* London: Department of Health.

— (2002*b*) *Models of Care for Substance Misuse Treatment.* London: Department of Health.

— & Social Services Inspectorate (1991) *Children in the Public Care.* London: HMSO.

— & — (1995) *The Challenge of Partnership in Child Protection: Practice Guide.* London: HMSO.

— & Welsh Office (1995) *Child Protection: Clarification of Arrangements Between the NHS and Other Agencies.* London: HMSO.

— & — (1999) *Mental Health Act 1983 Code of Practice.* London: Stationery Office.

—, British Medical Association & Conference of Medical Royal Colleges (1994) *Child Protection. Medical Responsibilities: Guidance for Doctors Working with Child Protection Agencies.* London: HMSO.

—, Home Office & Department for Education and Employment (1999) *Working Together to Safeguard Children.* London: Stationery Office.

Department of Health and Social Security (1975) *Better Services for the Mentally Ill.* London: HMSO.

— (1987) *Subject Access to Personal Health Information*. LAC (87) 10 HC. London: HMSO.

Dessent, T. (1996) *Meeting Special Educational Needs – Options for Partnership Between Health, Social and Education Services*. London: National Association for Special Educational Needs.

DeVaugh-Geiss, J., Moroz, G., Biederman, J., *et al* (1992) Clomipramine hydrochloride in childhood and adolescent obsessive–compulsive disorder – a multicenter trial. *Journal of the American Academy of Child and Adolescent Psychiatry*, **31**, 45–49.

Dische, S., Yule, W. & Corbett, J. (1983) Childhood nocturnal enuresis: factors associated with outcome of treatment with an enuretic alarm. *Developmental Medicine and Child Neurology*, **25**, 67–80.

Dolan, M., Holloway, J., Bailey, S., *et al* (1999) Health status of young offenders appearing before juvenile courts. *Journal of Adolescence*, **22**, 137–144.

Dungar, D., Pritchard, J., Hensman, S., *et al* (1986) The investigation of atypical psychosomatic illness: a team approach to diagnosis. *Clinical Pediatrics*, **25**, 341–344.

Dunn, J. (1996) Children's relationships: bridging the divide between cognitive and social development. *Journal of Child Psychology and Psychiatry*, **37**, 507–518.

Durkheim, E. (1970) *Suicide – A Study in Sociology*. London: Routledge & Keegan Paul.

— (1994) Childhood bereavement: consequences and therapeutic approaches. *Association of Child Psychology and Psychiatry Review and Newsletter*, **16**, 173–182.

Elizur, E. & Kaffman, M. (1983) Factors influencing the severity of childhood bereavement reactions. *American Journal of Orthopsychiatry*, **53**, 668–676.

Elliot, C. (1996) *British Ability Scales* (2nd edn) (BAS II). Windsor: NFER-Nelson.

Elmslie, G. J., Rush, A. J. & Weinburg, W. A. (1997) A double blind randomised placebo controlled trial of fluoxetine in children and adolescents with depression. *Archives of General Psychiatry*, **31**, 1031–1037.

Elton, A. (1988) Assessment of families for treatment. In *Child Sexual Abuse in the Family: Assessment and Treatment* (eds A. Bentovim, A. Elton, J. Hildebrand, *et al*), pp. 153–181. London: Wright.

Evans, M. O., Morgan, H. G., Hayward, A., *et al* (1999) Crisis telephone consultation for deliberate self-harm patients: effects on repetition. *British Journal of Psychiatry*, **175**, 23–27.

Evidence-Based Medicine Working Group (1992) Evidence-based medicine. A new approach to teaching the practice of medicine. *Journal of the American Medical Association*, **268**, 2420–2425.

Felce, D., Taylor, D. & Wright, K. (1994) People with learning disabilities. In *Healthcare Needs Assessment – The Epidemiology Based Needs Assessment Reviews, Vol. 2* (eds A. Stevens & J. Raffery), pp. 414–450. Oxford: Radcliffe Medical Press.

Feminist Review (1988) Family secrets: child sexual abuse. *Feminist Review*, special issue, spring.

Finkelhor, D. (1986) *A Sourcebook on Child Sexual Abuse*. Beverley Hills: Sage.

Fombonne, E. (1998) Interpersonal therapy for adolescent depression. *Child Psychology and Psychiatry Review*, **3**, 169–175.

Fonagy, P., Target, M., Cottrell, D., *et al* (2002) *What Works for Whom – A Critical Review of Treatments for Children and Adolescents*. London: Guilford Press.

Foreman, D. M. (2001) General practitioners and child and adolescent psychiatry: awareness and training of the new commissioners. *Psychiatric Bulletin*, **25**, 101–104.

Fox, C. & Joughin, C. (2002) *Childhood-Onset Eating Problems: Findings from Research*. London: Gaskell.

Gale, R. (1996) Managing a budget. In *Textbook of Management for Doctors* (ed. T. White), pp. 211–220. London: Churchill Livingstone.

Garralda, M. E. (1994) Primary care psychiatry. In *Child and Adolescent Psychiatry: Modern Approaches* (eds M. Rutter, E. Taylor & L. Hersov), pp. 1055–1070. Oxford: Blackwell Scientific.

Garrison, C. Z. (1989) The study of suicidal behavior in schools. *Suicide and Life-Threatening Behavior*, **19**, 120–130.

—, Lewinsohn, P. M., Marsteller, F., *et al* (1991) The assessment of suicidal behavior in adolescents. *Suicide and Life-Threatening Behavior*, **21**, 217–230.

Gatrell, J. (1996) Managing people. In *Textbook of Management for Doctors* (ed. T. White), pp. 127–134. London: Churchill Livingstone.

Geddes, J. (1999) Suicide and homicide by people with mental illness. *BMJ*, **318**, 1225–1226.

— & Harrison, P. J. (1997) Closing the gap between research and practice. *British Journal of Psychiatry*, **171**, 220–225.

Geist, R. (1977) Consultation on a pediatric surgical ward. *American Journal of Orthopsychiatry*, **47**, 432–444.

Gelder, M. (1999) Public attitudes to mental illness. Presentation to a meeting of the Royal College of Psychiatrists and the Royal Society of Medicine, quoted in Yamey, G. (1999) Young less tolerant of mentally ill than the old. *BMJ*, **319**, 1092.

General Medical Council (1995) *Confidentiality*. London: GMC.

— (1998*a*) *Maintaining Good Medical Practice*. London: GMC.

— (1998*b*) *Seeking Patients' Consent: The Ethical Considerations*. London: GMC.

— (1999) *Management in Health Care: The Role of Doctors*. London: GMC.

— (2000) *Revalidation*. London: GMC.

— (2001) *Good Medical Practice*. London: GMC.

George, C. (1996) A representational perspective of child abuse and internal working models of attachment and care giving. *Child Abuse and Neglect*, **20**, 411–424.

Gibbons, M. B. (1992) A child dies, a child survives: the impact of sibling loss. *Journal of Pediatric Health Care*, **6**, 65–72.

Gillance, H., Tucker, A., Aldridge, J., *et al* (1997) Bereavement: providing support for siblings. *Paediatric Nursing*, **9(5)**, 22–24.

Gillberg, C., Persson, E., Grufman, M., *et al* (1986) Psychiatric disorders in mildly and severely mentally retarded urban children and adolescents: epidemiological aspects. *British Journal of Psychiatry*, **149**, 68–74.

Goldberg, D. & Collier, P. (1999) Why are there so few adolescent day services? *Young Minds Magazine*, **40**, 14–15.

Goldstein, R. D., Wampler, N. S. & Wise, P. H. (1997) War experiences and distress symptoms of Bosnian children. *Pediatrics*, **100**, 873–878.

Goodman, R. (1998) *Child and Adolescent Mental Health Services: Reasoned Advice to Commissioners and Providers*. London: Institute of Psychiatry.

— (2001) The psychiatric properties of the strengths and difficulties questionnaire. *Journal of the American Academy of Child and Adolescent Psychiatry*, **40**, 1337–1345.

Goss, S. & Miller, C. (1995) *From Margin to Mainstream: Developing User and Carer Centred Community Care*. York: Joseph Rowntree Foundation.

Gostin, L. O. (2000) Human rights of persons with mental disabilities: the European Convention of Human Rights. *International Journal of Law and Psychiatry*, **23**, 125–159.

Gowers, S. G. & Shore, A. (2001) Development of weight and shape concerns in the aetiology of eating disorders. *British Journal of Psychiatry*, **179**, 236–242.

—, Wetman, J., Shore, A., *et al* (2000) Impact of hospitalisation on the outcome of adolescent anorexia nervosa. *British Journal of Psychiatry*, **176**, 138–141.

Graham, P. (1998) *Cognitive–Behaviour Therapy for Children and Families*. Cambridge: Cambridge University Press.

— (2000) Treatment interventions and findings from research: bridging the chasm in child psychiatry. *British Journal of Psychiatry*, **176**, 414–419.

Green, J. & Jacobs, B. (1998) *In-patient Child Psychiatry*. London: Routledge.

Green, K., Williams, C., Wright, B., *et al* (2001) Developing a child and adolescent mental health service for children with learning disabilities. *Psychiatric Bulletin*, **25**, 264–267.

Grizenko, N. & Papineau, D. (1992) A comparison of the cost-effectiveness of day treatment and residential treatment for children with severe behaviour problems. *Canadian Journal of Psychiatry*, **37**, 393–400.

Guyatt, G. H., Meade, M. O., Jaeschke, R. J., *et al* (2000) Practitioners of evidence based care. *BMJ*, **320**, 954–955.

Harding, J. (1999) Providing better services for mentally disordered offenders: pitfalls and prospects. *Probation Journal Special Issue – Working with Mentally Disordered Offenders*, **46**(2), 83–88.

Hardman, E. & Joughin, C. (1998) *FOCUS on Clinical Audit in Child and Adolescent Mental Health Services*. London: Gaskell.

Harrington, R. (1994) Affective disorders. In *Child and Adolescent Psychiatry: Modern Approaches* (eds M. Rutter, E. Taylor & L. Hersov), pp. 330–350. Oxford: Blackwell Scientific.

—— (1998) Clinically depressed adolescents. In *Cognitive–Behaviour Therapy for Children and Families* (ed. P. Graham), pp. 156–193. Cambridge: Cambridge University Press.

—— & Harrison, L. (1999) Unproven assumptions about the impact of bereavement on children. *Journal of the Royal Society of Medicine*, **92**, 230–233.

—— , Kerfoot, M., Dyer, E., *et al* (1998) Randomised trial of a home based family intervention for children who have deliberately poisoned themselves. *Journal of the American Academy of Child and Adolescent Psychiatry*, **37**, 512–518.

Harris, J. L., Westerby, M., Hill, T., *et al* (2001) User satisfaction: measurement and interpretation. *Journal of Family Planning and Reproductive Health Care*, **27**, 41–45.

Hatton, C. (1998) Intellectual disabilities: epidemiology and causes. In *Clinical Psychology and People with Intellectual Disabilities* (eds E. Emerson, C. Hatton, J. Bromley, *et al*), pp. 20–30. Chichester: John Wiley & Sons.

Hayter, J. (2000) Day therapy for adolescents: the evolution and practice of a day therapy service. *Young Minds Magazine*, **47**, 13–17.

Henggeler, S. W. (1999) Multi-systemic therapy: an overview of clinical procedures, outcomes and policy indications. *Child Psychology and Psychiatry Review*, **4**, 2–10.

——, Schoenwald, S. K., Bourduin, C. M., *et al* (1998) *Multisystemic treatment of antisocial behaviour in Children and Adolescents*. New York: Guilford Press.

Hewson, B. (2000) Why the Human Rights Act matters to doctors. *BMJ*, **321**, 780–781.

Hill, P. (1995) Committee practice. In *Management for Psychiatrists* (2nd edn) (eds D. Bhugra & A. Burns), pp. 248–261. London: Gaskell.

Hindley, P., Hill, P., McGuigan, P., *et al* (1994) Psychiatric disorder in deaf and hearing impaired children and young people: a prevalence study. *Journal of Child Psychology and Psychiatry*, **35**, 917–934.

Hinshaw, S. P., Owens, E. B., Wells, K. C., *et al* (2000) Family processes and treatment outcome in the MTA: negative/ineffective parenting practices in relation to multimodal treatment. *Journal of Abnormal Child Psychology*, **28**, 569–583.

HM Government (1998) *Tackling Drugs to Build a Better Britain. The Government's 10-year Strategy for Tackling Drug Misuse*. London: HMSO

HM Inspectorate of Prisons (1997) *Thematic Review of Young Prisoners*. London. Home Office.

HM Prison Service (1999) *Joint Prison Service/NHS Executive Working Party on the Future Organisation of Prison Health Care*. London: HMPS.

House of Commons Health Committee (1997) *Child and Adolescent Mental Health Services*. London: Stationery Office.

Home Office, Department of Health, Department of Education and Science & Welsh Office (1991) *Workign Together under the Children Act 1989: A Guide to Arrangements for Inter-Agency Cooperation for the Protection of Children from Abuse*. London: HMSO.

Howlin, P. (1994) Special educational treatment. In *Child and Adolescent Psychiatry: Modern Approaches* (eds M. Rutter, E. Taylor & L. Hersov), pp. 1071–1088. Oxford: Blackwell Scientific.

Huntley, M. (1996) *Griffiths Mental Developmental Scales from Birth to Two Years.* London: Association for Research on Infant and Child Development.

Hurry, J. & Storey, P. (2000) Assessing young people who deliberately harm themselves. *British Journal of Psychiatry,* **176**, 126–131.

Jasper, A., Smith, C. & Bailey, S. (1998) 100 girls in care referred to an adolescent forensic mental health service. *Journal of Adolescence,* **21**, 555–568.

Jellenik, M., Herzog, D. & Selter, F. (1981) A psychiatric consultation service for hospitalised children. *Psychosomatics,* **22**, 27–33.

Jenkins, J. M. & Smith, M. A. (1990) Factors protecting children living in dis-harmonious homes: maternal reports. *Journal of the American Academy of Child and Adolescent Psychiatry,* **29**, 60–69.

Joint College Working Party: Section for the Psychiatry of Mental Handicap and Child and Adolescent Psychiatry Section (1989) The training required to provide a psychiatric service for children and adolescents with mental handicap. *Psychiatric Bulletin,* **13**, 326–328.

Jones, D. P. H. (1992) *Interviewing the Sexually Abused Child. Investigation of Suspected Abuse.* London: Gaskell.

— & Ramchandani, P. (1999) *Child Sexual Abuse: Informing Practice from Research.* Abingdon: Radcliffe Medical.

Jones, E., Lucey, C. & Wadland, L. (2000) Triage: a waiting list initiative in a child mental health service. *Psychiatric Bulletin,* **24**, 57–59.

Joughin, C, & Zwi, M. (1999) *FOCUS on the Use of Stimulants in Children with Attention Deficit Hyperactivity Disorder: Evidence-Based Briefing.* London: Royal College of Psychiatrists Research Unit.

Junger-Tas, J. (1994) *Delinquent Behaviour Among Young People in the Western World.* Amsterdam: Kugler.

Kane, B. (1979) Children's concepts of death. *Journal of Genetic Psychology,* **134**, 141–153.

Kanner, L. (1943) Autistic disturbances of affective contact. *Nervous Child,* **2**, 217–250.

Kasper, J. & Nyamathi, A. (1988) Parents of children in the pediatric intensive care unit: what are their needs? *Heart and Lung,* **17**, 574–581.

Kazdin, A. E. (1995) *Conduct Disorder in Childhood and Adolescence.* London: Sage.

— (1997) Psychosocial treatments for conduct disorder. *Journal of Child Psychology and Psychiatry,* **38**, 161–178.

— (2000) Adolescent development, mental disorders, and decision making of delinquent youths. In *Youth on Trial. A Developmental Perspective on Juvenile Justice, Vol. 2* (eds T. Grisso & R. G. Shwartz), pp. 33–65. Chicago: Chicago University Press.

—, Siegal, T. & Bass, D. (1992) Cognitive problem solving skills and parent management training in the treatment of antisocial behaviours in children. *Journal of Consulting and Clinical Psychology,* **60**, 733–747.

Kelson, M. (1997) *User Involvement: A Guide to Developing Effective Strategies in the NHS.* London: College of Health.

Kendall, P. & Southam-Gerow, M. (1996) Long term follow up of a cognitive behavioural therapy for anxiety disordered youths. *Journal of Consulting and Clinical Psychology,* **64**, 724–730.

Kennedy, C. R. (1998) *A Guide for Purchasers of Tertiary Services for Children with Neurological Problems.* London: British Paediatric Neurology Association.

Kennedy, P. & Griffiths, H. (2000) *An Analysis of the Concerns of Consultant General Psychiatrists About Their Jobs, and of the Changing Practices That May Point Towards Solutions.* Durham: Northern Centre for Mental Health.

Kerfoot, M. (1988) Deliberate self-poisoning in childhood and early adolescence. *Journal of Child Psychology and Psychiatry,* **29**, 335–343.

—, Harrington, R. & Dyer, E. (1995) Brief home-based intervention with young suicide attempters and their families. *Journal of Adolescence,* **18**, 557–568.

—, Dyer, E., Harrington, V., *et al* (1996) Correlates and short-term course of self-poisoning in adolescents. *British Journal of Psychiatry*, **168**, 38–42.

Kiernan, C., & Kiernan, D. (1994) Challenging behaviour in schools for children with severe learning difficulties. *Mental Handicap Research*, **7**, 117–201.

Knapp, M. & Henderson, J. (1999) Health economic perspectives and evaluation of child and adolescent mental health services. *Current Opinions in Psychiatry*, **12**, 393–397.

Kolvin, I., Garside, R. F., Nicol, A. R., *et al* (1981) *Help Starts Here – The Maladjusted Child in the Ordinary School*. London: Tavistock.

Kraemer, S. (1994) *The Case for a Multidisciplinary Child and Adolescent Mental Health Community Service: The Liaison Model. A Guide for Managers, Purchasers and GPs*. London: Tavistock Clinic.

Kurtz, Z. (1992) *With Health in Mind: Mental Health Care for Children and Young People*. London: Action for Sick Children.

—, Thornes, R. & Wolkind, S. (1994) *Services for the Mental Health of Children and Young People in England: A National Review*. London: Maudsley Hospital and South Thames (West) Regional Health Authority.

—, Thornes, R. & Bailey, S. (1997) *Study of the Demands and Needs for Forensic Child and Adolescent Mental Health Services in England and Wales. Report to the Department of Health*. London: Department of Health.

Kyle, J. G. & Griggs, M. L. (1996) Deafness and mental health. In *Proceedings of International Congress of the Deaf (Tel Aviv 1995)*. Washington, MA: Gallaudet University Press.

Kyle, J. G. & Pullen, G. (1995) *Young Deaf People in Employment. Report to the Medical Research Council*. Bristol: CDS.

Lader, D., Singleton, N. & Meltzer, H. (2000) *Psychiatric Morbidity Among Young Offenders in England and Wales*. London: Office for National Statistics.

Land, T. (1997) *Services to Children and Young People Who Experience Emotional, Behavioural or Mental Health Problems in York and North Yorkshire: Multi-Agency Strategy*. York: North Yorkshire Health Authority.

Lask, B. (1987) Family therapy. *BMJ*, **294**, 203–204.

— (1994) Paediatric liaison work. In *Child and Adolescent Psychiatry: Modern Approaches* (eds M. Rutter, E. Taylor & L. Hersov), pp. 996–1005. Oxford: Blackwell Scientific.

— & Matthew, D. (1979) Childhood asthma – a controlled trial of family psycho-therapy. *Archives of Disease in Childhood*, **54**, 116–119.

Laugharne, R. (1999) Evidence-based medicine, user involvement and the post-modern paradigm. *Psychiatric Bulletin*, **23**, 641–643.

Leekam, S. R., Libby, S. J., Wing, L., *et al* (2002) The Diagnostic Interview for Social and Communication Disorders: algorithms for ICD–10 childhood autism and Wing and Gould autistic spectrum disorder. *Journal of Child Psychology and Psychiatry*, **43**, 327–342.

Lemouchoux, C., Millar, H. & Naji, S. (2001) Eating disorder in Scotland: starved of resources? *Psychiatric Bulletin*, **25**, 256–260.

Lerner, M. S. & Clum, G. A. (1990) Treatment of suicide ideators: a problem-solving approach. *Behavioral Therapy*, **21**, 403–411.

Leslie, S. A. (1992) Paediatric liaison. *Archives of Disease in Children*, **67**, 1046–1049.

Lewinsohn, P. M. & Clarke, G. N. (1990) Cognitive–behavioural treatment for depressed adolescents. *Behavioral Therapy*, **21**, 385–401.

Lilley, R., Lambden, P. & Newdick, C. (2001) *Understanding the Human Rights Act: A Tool Kit for the Health Service*. Oxford: Radcliffe Medical Press.

Linehan, M. M., Armstrong, H. E., Suarez, A., *et al* (1991) Cognitive behavioural treatment of chronically parasuicidal borderline patients. *Archives of General Psychiatry*, **48**, 1060–1064.

Little, M. & Mount, K. (1999) *Prevention and Early Intervention with Children in Need*. London: Action for Young People.

Lord, C., Rutter, M. & Le Couteur, A. (1994) Autism Diagnostic Interview – Revised: a revised version of a diagnostic interview for caregivers of individuals with possible pervasive developmental disorders. *Journal of Autism and Developmental Disorders*, **24**, 659–685.

—, Dilavore, P. C., Pickles, A., *et al* (2000) Autism Diagnostic Observation Schedule. A standard measure of social and communication deficits associated with the spectrum of autism. *Journal of Autism and Developmental Disorders*, **30**, 205–223.

Lovaas, O. (1987) Behavioural treatment and normal educational and intellectual functioning in young autistic children. *Journal of Consulting and Clinical Psychology*, **55**, 3–9.

March, J. (1995) Cognitive behavioral therapy for children and adolescents with O.C.D.: a review and recommendations for treatment. *Journal of the American Academy of Child and Adolescent Psychiatry*, **34**, 7–18.

Markantonakis, A. & Mathai, J. (1990) An evaluation of general practitioners' knowledge and satisfaction of a local child and family psychiatric service. *Psychiatric Bulletin*, **14**, 328–329.

Mason, R., Watts, E. & Hewison, J. (1995) Parental expectations of a child and adolescent psychiatric out-patient service. *ACPP Review and Newsletter*, **17**, 313–322.

Mattson, A. (1976) Child psychiatric ward rounds on pediatrics. *Journal of the American Academy of Child Psychiatry*, **15**, 357–365.

Maziade, M., Gingras, N., Bouchard, S., *et al* (1997) Long-term stability of diagnosis and symptom dimensions in a systematic sample of patients with onset of schizophrenia in childhood and early adolescence. II: Positive/negative distinction and childhood predictors of adult outcome. *British Journal of Psychiatry*, **169**, 371–378.

McClellan, J. & Werry, J. (1994) Practice parameters for the assessment and treatment of children and adolescents with schizophrenia. *Journal of the American Academy of Child and Adolescent Psychiatry*, **33**, 616–635.

McFadyen, A. (1999) Doubly disadvantaged: providing a psychotherapeutic and educational service to children with complex disorders and their families. *Clinical Child Psychology and Psychiatry*, **4**, 91–105.

McKay, I., & Hall, D. (1994) *Services for Children and Adolescents with Learning Disability (Mental Handicap)*. London: British Paediatric Association.

McLeavey, B. C., Daly, R. J., Ludgate, J. W., *et al* (1994) Interpersonal problem-solving skills training in the treatment of self-poisoning patients. *Suicide and Life-Threatening Behaviour*, **24**, 382–394.

Medical Research Council (2001) *Review of Autism Research, Epidemiology and Causes*. London: MRC.

Meltzer, H., Gatward, R., Goodman, R., *et al* (2000) *The Mental Health of Children and Adolescents in Great Britain*. London: National Statistics Office.

Mental Health Foundation (1997) *Don't Forget Us. Children with Learning Disabilities and Severe Challenging Behaviour. Report of a Committee Set up by the Mental Health Foundation*. London: Mental Health Foundation.

— (2002) *From Pregnancy to Early Childhood: Early Interventions to Enhance the Mental Health of Children and Families*. London: Mental Health Foundation.

Middleton, J. (2000) Applications in child mental health. *The Psychologist*, **13**, 27–29.

MIND (2001) *The Human Rights Act 1998*. London: MIND Publications.

Minuchin, S. (1974) *Families and Family Therapy*. London: Tavistock.

Mitchels, B. & Meadows, R. (1989) About courts. *BMJ*, **299**, 671–674.

Moran, G., Fonagy, P. & Kurtz, A. (1991) A controlled study of the psychoanalytic treatment of brittle diabetes. *Journal of the American Academy of Child and Adolescent Psychiatry*, **30**, 926–935.

Morgan, H. G., Jones, E. M. & Owen, J. H. (1993) Secondary prevention of non-fatal deliberate self-harm. The green card study. *British Journal of Psychiatry*, **163**, 111–112.

Morley, D. & Wilson, P. (2001) *Child and Adolescent Mental Health: Its Importance and How to Commission a Comprehensive Service. Guidance for Primary Care Trusts*. London: Young Minds.

Mortimore, P. (1995). The positive effects of schooling. In *Psychosocial Disturbances in Young People* (ed. M. Rutter), pp. 333–364. Cambridge: Cambridge University Press.

MTA Cooperative Group (1999) Moderators and mediators of treatment response for children with attention-deficit hyperactivity disorder. *Archives of General Psychiatry*, **56**, 1088–1096.

Mullen, P. E. (2000) Forensic mental health. *British Journal of Psychiatry*, **176**, 307–311.

Nadkarni, A., Parkin, A., Dogra, N., *et al* (2000) Characteristics of children and adolescents presenting to accident and emergency departments with deliberate self harm. *Emergency Medical Journal*, **17**, 98–102.

National Assembly for Wales (2001) *Child and Adolescent Mental Health Services: Everybody's Business*. Cardiff: Primary and Community Healthcare Division.

National Autistic Society (1983) *Consultation Response to the Health Select Committee Enquiry into Provision of NHS Mental Health Services*. London: NAS.

National In-Patient Child and Adolescent Psychiatry Study (NICAPS) (2001). *Key Findings of the Report Conference, 9 February 2001*. London: Royal College of Psychiatrists' Research Unit.

National Institute for Clinical Excellence (2000) *Guidance on the Use of Methylphenidate for Attention-Deficit Hyperactivity Disorder (ADHD) in Childhood*. London: National Health Service.

NHS Executive (1995) *Priorities and Planning Guidance for the NHS: 1997/98*. Leeds: NHSE.

—— (1998) *Signposts for Success in Commissioning and Providing Health Services for People with Learning Disabilities*. London: Department of Health.

—— (2001) *A Commitment to Quality, A Quest for Excellence: A Statement on Behalf of the Government, the Medical Profession and the NHS*. Leeds: NHS Executive.

NHS Health Advisory Service (1995a) *Together We Stand: The Commissioning, Role and Management of Child and Adolescent Mental Health Services*. London: HMSO.

—— (1995b) A strategic approach to commissioning and delivering child and adolescent mental health services. In *Together We Stand: The Commissioning, Role and Management of Child and Adolescent Services*, pp. 59–69. London: HMSO.

—— (1996) *The Substance of Young Needs: Children and Young People's Substance Misuse Services*. London: HMSO.

—— (1998) *Forging New Channels. Commissioning and Delivering Mental Health Services for People Who Are Deaf*. British Society for Mental Health and Deafness with permission of the Department of Health.

—— (2001) *The Substance of Young Needs*. Drugs Prevention Advisory Service. London: HMSO.

——, Mental Health Act Commission & Department of Health Social Services Inspectorate (1994) *A Review of the Adolescent Forensic Psychiatry Service Based on the Gardner Unit, Prestwick Hospital, Salford, Manchester*. London: NHS HAS.

Nicol, A. R. (1994) Practice in nonmedical settings. In *Child and Adolescent Psychiatry: Modern Approaches* (eds M. Rutter, E. Taylor & L. Hersov), pp. 1040–1054. Oxford: Blackwell Scientific.

Office of Population Censuses and Surveys (1989) *Surveys of Disability in Great Britain. Reports 1–6*. London: HMSO.

Oke, S. & Mayer, R. (1991) Referrals to child psychiatry – a survey of staff attitudes. *Archives of Disease in Childhood*, **66**, 862–865.

Oliver, C. (1995). Annotation. Self-injurious behaviour in children with learning disabilities: Recent advances in assessment and intervention. *Journal of Child Psychology and Psychiatry*, **30**, 900–927.

O'Neill-Byrne, K. & Browning, S. M. (1996) Which patients do GPs refer to which professional. *Psychiatric Bulletin*, **20**, 584–587.

Orford, E. (1998) Commentary on Kewley, G. D. (1998) Personal paper: attention deficit hyperactivity disorder is underdiagnosed and undertreated in Britain. *BMJ*, **316**, 1594–1596.

Outhwaite, W. (2000) *Implications of the Human Rights Act Upon Consent and Incapacity. From 'Incapacity and Consent' Conference*. London: IBC UK Conferences Limited.

Overmeyer, S. & Taylor, E. (1999) Annotation. Principles of treatment for hyperkinetic disorder: practice approaches for the U.K. *Journal of Child Psychology and Psychiatry*, **40**, 1147–1157.

Oxman, A., Sackett, D. L. & Guyatt, G. H. (1993) Users' guides to the medical literature. 1: How to get started. The Evidence-Based Medicine Working Group. *JAMA*, **270**, 2093–2095.

Park, M., Langa, A., Likierman, H., *et al* (1991) Setting up a new regional child and family psychiatry unit: the involvement of referrers. *Psychiatric Bulletin*, **15**, 142–144.

Partridge, I., Redmond, C., Williams, C., *et al* (1999) Evaluating family therapy in a child and adolescent mental health service. *Psychiatric Bulletin*, **23**, 531–533.

Partridge, I., Casswell, G. & Richardson, G. (2001) Assessing the risks posed by parents. *Child Psychology and Psychiatry Review*, **6**, 110–113.

Pearson, G. (1983) *Hooligans: A History of Respectable Fears*. London: Macmillan Education.

Peckham, M. (1991) *Research for Health: A Research and Development Strategy for the N.H.S.* London: Department of Health.

Pelham, W. E. & Bender, M. (1982) Peer interactions of hyperactive children: assessment and treatment. In *Advances in Learning and Behaviour Difficulties* (eds K. Gradow & I. Gialer). Greenwich, CT: JI Press.

Pelham, W. E., Carlson, C., Sams, S. E., *et al* (1993) Separate and combined effects of methylphenidate and behavior modification on boys with attention deficit hyperactivity disorder in the classroom. *Journal of Consulting and Clinical Psychology*, **61**, 506–515.

Pennels, M., Smith, S. & Poppleton, R. (1992) Bereavement and adolescents: a groupwork approach. *Association of Child Psychiatry and Psychology Newsletter*, **14**, 173–178.

Pettite, D. B. (1994) *Meta-analysis, Decision Analysis and Cost Effectiveness Analysis*. Oxford: Oxford University Press.

Pettle-Michael, S. A. & Lansdown, R. G. (1986) Adjustment to the death of a sibling. *Archives of Disease in Childhood*, **61**, 278–283.

Pfeffer, C. R., Carus, D., Seigel, K., *et al* (2000) Child survivors of parental death from cancer or suicide: depressive and behavioural outcomes. *Psycooncology*, **9**, 1–10.

Place, M., Rajah, S. & Crake, T. (1990) Combining day patient treatment with family work in a child psychiatry clinic. *European Archives of Psychiatry and Neurological Science*, **239**, 373–378.

Pollock, G. H. (1986) Childhood sibling loss. A family tragedy. *Pediatric Annals*, **15**, 851–855.

Quality Network for In-Patient CAMHS (2001) *QNIC – Quality Network for In-Patient CAMHS: Service Standards*. London: Royal College of Psychiatrists' Research Unit.

Reder, P., Lucey, C. & Fellow-Smith, E. (1994) Surviving cross examination in court. *Journal of Forensic Psychiatry*, **4**, 489–496.

Richardson, G. & Cottrell, D. (2003) Service innovations: second opinions in child and adolescent psychiatry. *Psychiatric Bulletin*, **27**, 22–24.

— & Harris-Hendricks, J. (1996) Ethical and legal issues: (a) Confidentiality, consent and the courts. In *Child and Adolescent Psychiatry. A New Century* (eds J. Harris-Hendricks & M. Black), pp. 40–43 (Occasional Paper OP33). London: Royal College of Psychiatrists.

— & Partridge, I. (2000) Child and adolescent mental health services: liaison with tier 1 services. A consultation exercise with school nurses. *Psychiatric Bulletin*, **24**, 462–463.

—, Foxton, T. & Cross, M. (1998) Section E – Documentation. In *Focus on Clinical Audit in Child and Adolescent Mental Health Services* (eds E. Hardman & C. Joughin), pp. 73–77. London: Gaskell.

Richardson, W. S. (1996) Evidence based medicine: what it is and what it isn't. *BMJ*, **312**, 71–72.

Rifkin, S. B., Lewando-Hunt, G. & Draper, A. K. (2000) *Participatory Approaches in Health Promotion and Health Planning: A Literature Review*. London: Health Development Agency.

Roberts, S. & Partridge, I. (1998) Allocation of referrals within a child and adolescent mental health service. *Psychiatric Bulletin*, **22**, 487–489.

—, Foxton, T., Partridge, I., *et al* (1998) Establishing a specialist eating disorders team. *Psychiatric Bulletin*, **22**, 214–216.

Rosenberg, W. & Donald, A. (1995) Evidence-based medicine: an approach to clinical problem solving. *BMJ*, **310**, 1122–1125.

Rotherham, M. J. (1987) Evaluation of imminent danger for suicide among youth. *American Journal of Orthopsychiatry*, **57**, 102–110.

Royal College of Psychiatrists (1982) The management of parasuicide in young people under 16. *Bulletin of the Royal College of Psychiatrists*, **6**, 182–185.

— (1992*a*) *Eating Disorders* (Council Report CR14). London: Royal College of Psychiatrists.

— (1992*b*) *Psychiatric Services for Children and Adolescents with Mental Handicap* (Council Report CR17). London: Royal College of Psychiatrists.

— (1998) *Managing Deliberate Self Harm in Young People* (Council Report CR64). London: Royal College of Psychiatrists.

— (1999*a*) *Offenders with Personality Disorder* (Council Report CR71). London: Royal College of Psychiatrists.

— (1999*b*) *Guidance on Staffing of Child and Adolescent In-patient Psychiatry Units* (Council Report CR76). London: Royal College of Psychiatrists.

— (2000) *Good Psychiatric Practice 2000* (Council Report CR83). London: Royal College of Psychiatrists.

— (2001) *Good Psychiatric Practice: CPD* (Council Report CR90). London: Royal College of Psychiatrists.

Royal College of Psychiatrists' Research Unit (2001) *Clinical Governance Standards for Mental Health and Learning Disability Services*. London: Royal College of Psychiatrists' Research Unit.

Russell, G., Szmukler, G. I., Dare, C., *et al* (1987) An evaluation of family therapy in anorexia nervosa and bulimia nervosa. *Archives of General Psychiatry*, **44**, 1047–1056.

Russell, P. (1996) Issues arising from the implementation of the Code of Practice on the Identification and Assessment of Special Educational Needs. *Child Psychology and Psychiatry Review*, **1**, 110–111.

Rutter, M. (1981) *Maternal Deprivation Reassessed*. London: Penguin.

— (1985) Resilience in the face of adversity: protective factors and resilience to psychiatric disorder. *British Journal of Psychiatry*, **147**, 598–611.

— (1987) Psychosocial resilience and protective mechanisms. *American Journal of Orthopsychiatry*, **57**, 316–331.

— (1990) Psychosocial resilience and protective factors. In *Risk and Protective Factors in the Development of Psychopathology* (eds J. Rolf, A. S. Masten, D. Cichetti, *et al*), pp. 181–214. Cambridge: Cambridge University Press.

— (1999) Psychosocial adversity and child psychopathology. *British Journal of Psychiatry*, **174**, 480–493.

— & Smith, D. J. (1995) *Psychosocial Disorders in Young People: Time Trends and their Causes*. Chichester: John Wiley & Sons.

—, Graham, P. & Yule, W. (1970) *A Neuropsychiatric Study in Childhood*. London: Heinemann/Spastic International Medical Publications.

—, Maughan, B., Mortimore, P., *et al* (1979) *Fifteen Thousand Hours*. London: Open Books.

—, Giller, H. & Hagell, A. (1998) *Antisocial Behaviour by Young People*. Cambridge: Cambridge University Press.

Sackett, D., Rosenberg, W. M. C., Gray, J. A. M., *et al* (1997) *Evidence-Based Medicine. How to Practice and Teach E.B.M*. London: Churchill Livingstone.

Sainsbury Centre for Mental Health (2000) *An Executive Briefing on the Implications of the Human Rights Act 1998 for Mental Health Services*. London: Sainsbury Centre for Mental Health.

Salkovskis, P. M., Atha, C. & Storer, D. (1990) Cognitive–behavioural problem solving in the treatment of patients who repeatedly attempt suicide. A controlled trial. *British Journal of Psychiatry*, **157**, 871–876.

Sanders, M. R., Sheherd, R.W. & Cleghorn, G. (1994) The treatment of abdominal pain in children: a controlled comparison of cognitive–behavioural family intervention and standard paediatric care. *Journal of Consulting and Clinical Psychology*, **62**, 306–314.

Scally, G. & Donaldson, L. J. (1998) Clinical governance and the drive for quality improvement in the new NHS in England. *BMJ*, **317**, 61–65.

Schmidt, U. (1998) Eating disorders and obesity. In *Cognitive–Behaviour Therapy for Children and Families* (ed. P. Graham), pp. 262–281. Cambridge: Cambridge University Press.

— (2001) Eating disorder services: starved of resources. *Psychiatric Bulletin*, **25**, 241–242.

— & Treasure, J. (1993) *Getting Better Bit(e) by Bit(e)*. Englewood Cliffs, NJ: Lawrence Erlbaum.

Schopler, E. (1997) Implementation of TEACHH philosophy. In *Handbook of Autism and Pervasive Developmental Disorders* (eds D. Cohen & F. Volkmar), pp. 767–795. New York: John Wiley & Sons.

—, Richler, R. & Renner, B. (1986) *The Childhood Autism Rating Scale (CARS) for Diagnostic Screening and Classification of Autism*. New York: Irvington.

Schotte, D. E. & Clum, G. A. (1987) Problem-solving skills in suicidal psychiatric patients. *Journal of Consulting and Clinical Psychology*, **55**, 49–54.

Schwamm, J. S. & Maloney, M. J. (1997) Developing a psychiatry study group for community paediatricians. *Journal of the American Academy of Child and Adolescent Psychiatry*, **36**, 706–708.

Scott, S. (1998) Aggressive behaviour in childhood. *BMJ*, **316**, 202–206.

Shapiro, E. S., Shapiro, A. K. & Funop, G. (1989) Controlled study of haloperidol, pimozide and placebo for the treatment of Gilles de la Tourette syndrome. *Archives of General Psychiatry*, **46**, 722–730.

Shepherd, J. P. & Farrington, B. P. (1996) The prevention of delinquency with particular reference to violent crime. *Medicine, Science and the Law*, **36**, 331–336.

Shipman, M. D. (1968) *Sociology of the School*, pp. 13–14. London: Longman.

Shoebridge, P. J. & Gowers, S. G. (2000) Parental high concern and adolescent-onset anorexia nervosa. A case–control study to investigate direction of causality. *British Journal of Psychiatry*, **176**, 132–137.

SIGN (1997) *Mental Health Services for Deaf People: Are They Appropriate?* Buckinghamshire: SIGN.

Silveira, W.R. (1991) *Consultation in Residential Care*. Aberdeen: Aberdeen University Press.

Silverman, P. R. & Worden, J. W. (1992) Children's reactions in the early months after the death of a parent. *American Journal of Orthopsychiatry*, **62**, 93–104.

—, Nickman, S. & Worden, J. W. (1992) Detachment revisited. The child's reconstruction of a dead parent. *American Journal of Orthopsychiatry*, **62**, 494–503.

Skynner, A. C. R. (1976) *One Flesh; Separate Persons*. London: Constable.

Skynner, R. & Cleese, J. (1994) *Life and How To Survive It*. London: Mandarin.

Smith, J., Wheeler, J. & Bone, D. (2001) Anarchy and assessment of complex families: order not disorder. *Clinical Child Psychology and Psychiatry*, **6**, 605–608.

Smith, P., Perrin, S. & Yule, W. (1998) Post-traumatic stress disorders. In *Cognitive–Behaviour Therapy for Children and Families* (ed. P. Graham), pp. 127–142. Cambridge: Cambridge University Press.

Smith, S. C. & Pennels, M. (1995) *Interventions with Bereaved Children*. London: Jessica Kingsley.

Sparrow, S. (1997) Developmentally based assessment. In *Handbook of Autism and Pervasive Developmental Disorders* (ed. D. Cohen & F. Volkmar), pp. 411–477. New York: John Wiley & Sons.

—, Balla, D. & Cicchetti, D. (1984) *Vineland Adaptive Behavior Scales*. Pine Circles, MN: American Guidance Service.

Stein, L. & Jabaley, T. (1981) Early identification and parent counselling. In *Deafness and Mental Health* (ed. L. Stein). New York: Grune and Stratton.

Strauss, G., Chassin, M. & Lock, J. (1995) Can experts agree when to hospitalize adolescents? *Journal of the American Academy of Child and Adolescent Psychiatry*, **34**, 418–424.

Sturge, J. (1989) Joint work in paediatrics: a child psychiatry perspective. *Archives of Disease in Childhood*, **64**, 155–158.

Subotski, F. & Berelowitz, M. (1990) Consumer views at a child guidance clinic. *Newsletter of the Association for Child Psychology and Psychiatry*, **12**, 8–12.

Thompson, A. & Place, M. (1995) What influences general practitioners' use of child psychiatry services? *Psychiatric Bulletin*, **19**, 10–12.

Thorin, E., Yovanoff, P. & Irvin, L. (1996) Dilemmas faced by families during their young adults transitions to adulthood: a brief report. *Mental Retardation*, **34**, 117–120.

Treasure, J. & Schmidt, V. (2001) Ready, willing and able to change: motivational aspects of the assessment and treatment of eating disorders. *European Eating Disorders Review*, **9**, 4–18.

Tuffnell, G. (1993) Psychiatric court reports in child care cases: what constitutes good practice? *ACPP Review and Newsletter*, **15**, 219–224.

—, Cottrell, D. & Giorgiades, D (1996) Good practice for expert witnesses. *Clinical Child Psychology and Psychiatry*, **3**, 365–385.

Tutt, N. (1995) Transitions – children with disabilities and their passage into adulthood. *Social Information Systems Management Update*, **1**, 44–56.

Van Eerdewegh, M. M., Clayton, P. J. & Van Eerdewegh, P. (1985) The bereaved child: variables influencing early psychopathology. *British Journal of Psychiatry*, **147**, 188–194.

Vandvik, I. H. (1994) Collaboration between child psychiatry and paediatrics: the state of the relationship in Norway. *Acta Paediatrica*, **83**, 884–887.

Vikan, A. (1985) Psychiatric epidemiology in a sample of 1510 ten year old children. *Journal of Child Psychology and Psychiatry*, **76**, 55–75.

Vizard, E. & Harris, P. (1997) *The Expert Witness Pack*. Bristol: Family Law

—& Usiskin, J. (1999) Providing individual psychotherapy for young sexual abusers of other children. In *Children and Young People Who Sexually Abuse Others: Challenges and Responses* (eds M. Erooga & H. Massen). London: Routledge.

Voeller, K. K. (1991) Clinical management of attention deficit hyperactivity disorder. *Journal of Child Neurology*, **6** (suppl.), S51–S67.

Wallace, S. A., Crown, J. M., Cox, A. D., *et al* (1995) *Epidemiologically Based Needs Assessment: Child and Adolescent Mental Health*. London: Department of Health.

Ward, A., Ramsay, R. & Treasure, J. (1995) Eating disorders: not such a slim speciality? *Psychiatric Bulletin*, **19**, 723–724.

Wasserman, A. L. (1988) Helping families get through the holidays after the death of a child. *American Journal of Diseases in Childhood*, **142**, 1284–1286.

Wechsler, D. (1991) *Wechsler Intelligence Scale for Children* (3rd edn) (WISC III). San Antonio, TX: Psychological Corporation.

Weddell-Monnig, J. & Lumley, J. (1980) Child deafness and mother–child interaction. *Child Development*, **51**, 766–774.

Weeramanthri, T. & Keaney, F. (2000) What do inner city general practitioners want from a child and adolescent mental health service? *Psychiatric Bulletin*, **24**, 258–260.

Weiner, A., Withers, K., Patrick, M., *et al* (1999) What changes are of value in severely disturbed children? *Clinical Child Psychology and Psychiatry*, **4**, 201–213.

Weiss, G. (1996) Attention deficit hyperactivity disorder. In *Child and Adolescent Psychiatry* (ed. M. Lewis), pp. 544–565. Baltimore, MD: Williams and Wilkins.

Wells, K. C., Pelham, W. E., Kotrein, R. A., *et al* (2001) Psychosocial treatment strategies in the MTA study: rationale, methods and critical issues in design and implementation. *Journal of Abnormal Child Psychology*, **28**, 483–505.

Whalen, C. K., Henker, B. & Hinshaw, S. B. (1985) Cognitive behavioural therapies for hyperactive children: premises, problems and prospects. *Journal of Abnormal Child Psychology*, **13**, 391–410.

Wheeler, J., Bone, D. & Smith, J. (1998) Whole day assessments: a team approach to complex multi-problem families. *Clinical Child Psychology and Psychiatry*, **3**, 169–181.

Will, D. (1989) Feminism, child sexual abuse and the (long overdue) demise of systems mysticism. *Context*, **9**, 12–15.

Williams, C., Wright, B. & Smith, R. (1999*a*) CHEAF (Child Health and Education Assesment Forum): a multidisciplinary pow-wow for children. *Psychiatric Bulletin*, **23**, 104–106.

—, Wright, B. & Partridge, I. (1999*b*) Attention deficit hyperactivity disorder – a review. *British Journal of General Practice*, **49**, 563–571.

—, —, Callaghan, G., *et al* (2003) Do children with autism learn to read more readily by computer assisted instruction or traditional book methods? A pilot study. *Autism* (in press).

Williams, J. (1983) Teaching how to counsel in a pediatric clinic. *Journal of the American Academy of Child Psychiatry*, **22**, 399–403.

Williams, R. (1992) *A Concise Guide to the Children Act 1989*. London: Gaskell.

Williamson, C. (1992) *Whose Standards? Consumer and Professional Standards in Health Care*. Buckingham: Open University Press.

Wilson, E. & Waters, J. (1997) *Developing Links with Primary Care: A Report on the One Year Project for the Division of Child and Family Mental Health*. South Tees Community and Mental Health NHS Trust.

Wilson, G., Eldredge, K. L. & Smith, D. (1991) Cognitive behavioural treatment of bulimia nervosa: a controlled evaluation. *Behaviour Research and Therapy*, **29**, 579–583.

Wing, L. & Gould, J. (1979) Severe impairments of social interaction and associated abnormalities in children: epidemiology and classification. *Journal of Autism and Childhood Schizophrenia*, **9**, 11–29.

—, Leekam, S. R., Libby, S. J., *et al* (2002) The Diagnostic Interview for Social and Communication Disorders: background inter-rater reliability and clinical use. *Journal of Child Psychology and Psychiatry*, **43**, 307–325.

Wolkind, S. (1994) Legal aspects of child care. In *Child and Adolescent Psychiatry: Modern Approaches* (eds M. Rutter, E. Taylor & L. Hersov), pp. 1089–1102. Oxford: Blackwell Scientific.

Wolpert, M., Fuggle, P., Cottrell, D., *et al* (2002) *Drawing on the Evidence*. Leicester: British Psychological Society.

World Health Organization (1992) *The ICD–10 Classification of Mental and Behavioural Disorders*. Geneva: WHO.

Wright, B. & Partridge, I. (1999). Speaking ill of the dead. *Clinical Child Psychology and Psychiatry*, **4**, 225–231.

Wright, B., Williams, C. & Partridge, I. (1999) Management advice for children with chronic fatigue syndrome: a systematic study of information from the internet. *Irish Journal of Psychological Medicine*, **16**(2), 67–71.

—, Partridge, I. & Williams, C. (2000) Evidence and attribution: reflections upon the management of attention deficit hyperactivity disorder (ADHD). *Clinical Child Psychology and Psychiatry*, **5**, 626–636.

Wright, J. B., Aldridge, J., Gillance, H., *et al* (1996) Hospice based groups for bereaved siblings. *European Journal of Palliative Care*, **3**, 10–15.

Young Minds (1996) *Mental Health in Your School: A Guide for Teachers and Schools*. London: Jessica Kingsley.

Zimet, S. G., Farley, G. K. & Zimet, G. D. (1994) Home behaviours of children in three treatment settings: an out-patient clinic, a day hospital, and an inpatient hospital. *Journal of the American Academy of Child and Adolescent Psychiatry*, **33**, 56–59.

Index

Compiled by Linda English

administrative staff 18
adolescent forensic mental health teams 182
alcohol misuse *see* drug and alcohol teams
annual budget 19
anxiety management 42
area child protection committee (ACPC) 31, 33
Asperger's syndrome 142, 149
attachment 163, 175
attentional problems services 150–156
  assessment 152–154
  and child health services 152
  and family attributions 152, 153, 154
  intervention 154–156
  medication 100, 154–156
  nature of service 151–152
  psychosocial interventions 152, 156
attention-deficit hyperactivity disorder (ADHD) 100, 111, 150–156, 181
audit and evaluation 22, 25, 51, 115–116, 129–130, 140–141, 166
autistic spectrum disorders (ASD) services 142–149
  establishing a service 146–147
  information for families 148
  interventions 148–149
  and learning disabilities services 131, 136–137, 146
  organisation of assessment 144–146
  and paediatric liaison 111
  referrals to multi-disciplinary forum 145–146
  and respite 118
  screening 147
  training 147–148

behavioural management 137, 139
behavioural therapies 52, 100–101, 156
bereavement services 161–166
  audit and evaluation 166
  functions of team 162
  indications for bereavement work 161
  interventions 165
  managing bereavement 162–163
  multi-agency groups 165–166
  networking 163–164
  planning and training 164
  team membership 164

CAMHS learning disability teams 134–135, 136, 137–138, 139
CAMHS management teams 19
Care Programme Approach 122
caring for professionals 4–5
case work 99–100
Checklist for Autism in Toddlers 147
child, adolescent and family psychiatrists 43–44
child abuse and neglect 8, 30–33, 167, 174–177
child protection 30–33, 74
  and bereavement services 162
  inter-agency cooperation 32–33
  and paediatric liaison 111
  parenting risk assessment services 174–177
  and social workers 44
  suspicion and disclosure of abuse or neglect 31
child psychotherapists 101
Children Act 1989: 5, 27–28, 31, 44, 68, 69, 179
clinical child psychologists 43
clinical decision making 47–49
clinical directors 41
clinical effectiveness 50–51
clinical governance 21–26, 61
  annual reports 24–26
  definition 21
  and in-patient psychiatric care 124
  objectives 21
  requirements 22–24
cognitive therapy 101

commissioning 11–12
community mental health workers 78
community psychiatric nurses (CPNs) 9,
   43
comorbidity 51
competence 34–35
   assessment 35
   Gillick competence 30, 34
conduct disorder 119, 180
confidentiality 31, 37, 57, 58, 83
consent 29–30, 33–35
   and competence 34–35
   definition 33–34
   and Human Rights Act 1998: 37
   and in-patient care 30, 124–125
consultant psychiatrists 39, 40–42, 43–44,
   121
consultation *see* liaison and consultation
containment 100
context of CAMHS 7–15
continuing professional development
   (CPD) 22, 61
coordination of team 24
cost-effectiveness 50–51
counselling 101–102, 139
county courts 69
court reports 66–74
   charging 69–70
   civil matters 67
   court appearances 71–73
   criminal matters 67
   gathering information 70–71
   level of court 69
   and medical members of CAMHS 70
   and non-medical members of CAMHS
      70
   and parenting risk assessment services
      175, 176
   preparation 71
   professional *v.* expert witnesses 66–67
   questions to be answered 68
   requests and agreement between parties
      68
   requests from solicitors 66
   time-scale for preparation 68
   training issues 73–74
   treatment recommendations 67
crack cocaine 170
creative therapies 102
Crime and Disorder Act 1998: 67, 179
Crown Court 69
current initiatives 11–12

day patient services 112–116
   evaluation 115–116
   provision and organisation 112–114
   staffing 114–115
deaf children 105
deliberate self-harm 126–130
   assessment and management 127–128

in-patient psychiatric care 123
intervention and follow-up 128–129
in parents or carers 129
recording 129–130
service provision 127
teaching and training on management
   130
urgent referrals 93
and youth offending 181, 183
disciplinary autonomy 39
documentation 37, 108, 129–130
drug action teams (DATs) 169
drug and alcohol action teams (DAATs)
   169
drug and alcohol teams 167–173
   at-risk groups 167–168
   need for services 167–168
   provision 170–172
   service responses 169–170
   strategic planning process 168–169
   treatment aims 171
drug overdoses 93
drug treatments 100, 154–156

early intervention programmes 53
eating disorders services 157–160
   initial assessment 159
   in-patient care 120, 121, 123, 124,
      159–160
   intervention 101, 159–160
   referral 159
   specialist service integrated with locality
      CAMHS 157–158
economics 8–9, 50–51
educational psychologists 153–154
educational staff, liaison with 85–86, 89,
   153–154
emergencies 93, 118, 123
empowerment of service users 59
ENB 603 course 43, 65, 122, 170
European Convention on Human Rights
   (ECHR) 35–37
evidence-based practice 5, 12, 46–54, 189
   access to evidence 22, 46–47
   and CAMHS 51–52, 99
   and child and family preferences 48
   clinical effectiveness and cost-
      effectiveness 50–51
   and clinical practice 47–49
   critical appraisal 49
   evidence-based resources 49–50
   and external clinical evidence 47
   and individual clinical expertise 48, 49
   and in-patient psychiatric care 123
   issues in practice 52–54
   randomised controlled trials 51
expert witnesses 66–74

Family Division of High Court 69
family therapy 102–105, 159

forensic services 178–184
  adolescent forensic mental health teams
    182
  background 179–180
  comorbid factors with offending
    180–181
  definitions 178–179
  and female adolescents 181, 183
  four-tier model 183–184
  peripatetic outreach teams 184
  problem profiles 180–181
  requirements of young offenders
    181–182
  routes into offending 180
  strategic framework 183–184
  Tier 4 centres of specialist expertise 184
  and young people in prison 179–180,
    182–183
further education establishments, links
  with 65
future directions 14–15
general practitioners 25–26, 83, 88, 89, 91

Gillick competence 30, 34

health care records 37
health service management, focus on 9
health visitors 78–79, 147
heroin 167, 170–172
hierarchy of regard 87
High Court 69
homelessness 181
host organisation 19, 20, 190
Human Rights Act 1998 (HRA) 33, 35–37

individual development reviews (IDRs) 22
individual psychotherapy 101
information technology 22
innovation 23
in-patient psychiatric care 117–125
  adequacy of provision 120
  admission criteria 117, 118, 119–120, 125
  alternatives 121
  catchment areas 119, 121
  contractual commitment to
    commissioning authority 121
  and day patient services 113
  detention under Mental Health Act
    29–30, 44, 123
  discharge planning 119, 121–122, 123
  for eating disorders 120, 124, 159–160
  effectiveness of provision 120
  future agenda 125
  increasing awareness of service 121
  and integration between tiers 4
  integration into continuum of care 119
  and key worker/primary nurse system
    122
  organisational issues 121–125
  for pre-pubertal children 123, 125

  purpose 117–119
  and substance misuse 119, 123, 171–172
  and Tier 4 link workers 124
in-patient psychiatric nurses 43, 122, 125
integration between tiers 3–4
integration of organisational structure 4
intensive-care teams 121
inter-agency collaboration/cooperation 2, 8,
  9
  and child protection 32–33
  and national policy 12, 88
  and paediatric liaison 110–111
  and referral management 93–94
  and training 61, 63–64
  and treatment 99–100
internet access 63

joint-agency social care organisations 12

leadership 41–42
learning disabilities services 131–141
  allocation of resources 132
  assessment process 138
  and autistic spectrum disorders 131,
    136–137, 146
  CAMHS learning disability teams
    134–135, 136, 137–138, 139
  consultation and liaison 139
  establishing new service 135
  evaluation 140–141
  and historical situation 132
  intervention 138–139
  management structure of provider 133
  organisation 132
  referral process 136–137
  role of team 137–138
  service considerations 132–135
  strategies for work load management
    133
  teaching and training 140
  team structure 136
  transition to adult services 139–140
legislation 27–37
liaison and consultation
  and bereavement services 162, 163
  and learning disabilities services 139
  and paediatric services see paediatric
    liaison
  with Tier 1 professionals 79, 82–90
    challenges to 82–84
    and confidentiality 83
    effectiveness of interventions 84
    establishment of forum for liaison 89
    evaluation of consultation 84–85
    future agenda 88–89
    and ignorance of other agencies'
      involvement 83
    liaison with educational staff 85–86
    liaison with primary care services
      87–88

liaison and consultation with
    Tier 1 professionals, cont'd
    liaison with social services
      departments 87
    and national policy 88
    and poor management of CAMHS
      83–84
    and primary mental health workers 89
    principles of consultation 84–85
    and protocols for assessment of
      mental health problems 89
    and referral system 82–83
    and relationships 85
    and resources 83, 88–89
    and sectorisation 93
    and stigma 84
    and teacher training 89
libraries 63

magistrates' courts 69
management 16–20
  CAMHS management team 19
  and clinical governance 21, 24
  and liaison/consultation with Tier 1
    83–84
  problems 7–9
  roles 18, 41
  of site 19
  supportive and effective 24
  in tiers 17
  within host organisation 20
media responses to children's behaviour 7
medical negligence 71
medical responsibility 41, 44, 190
medication 100, 154–156
mental disorders 40, 75, 190
Mental Health Act 1983: 27, 28–30
  and consent 33–34
  detention under 29–30, 44, 123
mental health problems 40, 75, 190
mental health promotion 77, 79–80
motivational enhancement therapy 101
multi-agency working *see* inter-agency
  collaboration/cooperation
multi-disciplinary working 2, 17–18,
    38–45
  and attentional problems services 150, 151
  and clinical governance 23
  and day patient services 114
  and evidence-based practice 54
  and in-patient psychiatric care 122
  and learning disabilities services 136
  and neuropsychology services 186
  and paediatric liaison 109
  and parenting risk assessment services
    174, 175
  and referrals 95
  role adequacy 40, 44
  role legitimacy 40–42
  roles of individual disciplines 43–45

  role support 42
  tensions 38
  and training 61, 62, 63
multi-systemic therapy 181

National Service Framework for Children
  11
National Treatment Agency 168
neuropsychology and neuropsychiatry
    services 185–188
  and age effects 186
  assessment 187–188
  difference between adults and children
    185–186
  establishing a service 185–187
  interventions 188
  links with other professionals 186–187
  multi-disciplinary team 186
The New NHS 11

organisation 3–4, 16–20
outcomes
  and economics 8–9
  and evidence-based practice 54

paediatric liaison 107–111
  and attentional problems services 151
  cooperation and mutual respect 110
  effects of liaison team 109–111
  establishing liaison team 108
  joint working 110
  medical member of team 109
  multi-agency assessment 111
  in other settings 111
  and referrals 109–110
  and self-harm 130
  structure of liaison team 109
  urgent cases 110
paediatric ward care 121, 123, 124
paramountcy principle 54
parental consent 30, 34
parenting risk assessment services
    174–177
  assessment process 176–177
  and developmental context 175
  and forensic context 175
  management of referrals 175–176
  multi-disciplinary perspectives 175
  professional meetings 176
  and systems theory 175
  team philosophy 175
  team structure 175
parent support and management 97–99
personal development plans (PDPs) 62
personality disorder 181
political context 11–12
prevention 52–53
primary care services
  commissioning by 11–12
  liaison with 87–88

primary mental health workers 83, 88
  and family therapy 103
  and future agenda 89
  objectives 79–80
  and referrals 76, 78, 81, 93
  requirements for effective functioning
    81
  role 78
principles guiding service delivery 2–6
prioritisation 25–26, 52, 91, 92
prisons, mental health care in 179–180,
  182–183
professional regulation 23
professional witnesses 66–74
protocols for assessment of mental health
  problems 89
psychiatrists 39, 40–42, 43–44, 92, 121,
  127
psychopharmacological treatments 100,
  154–156
psychosomatic problems 110, 111, 120,
  124
psychotherapy 101
psychotic disorders 120, 123, 181

quality of care see clinical governance

randomised controlled trials (RCTs) 51
referrals 3, 12
  allocation meetings 92
  and anxiety of referrer 76, 82–83
  awareness of context 95
  to bereavement services 162
  clarification 93
  and co-working 95
  to day patient services 114
  and disciplinary function 94
  to eating disorders services 159
  for family therapy 103
  and individual work loads 94
  inter-agency work 93–94
  to learning disabilities services
    136–137
  management 91–95
  and medical responsibility 41
  to paediatric liaison teams 109–110
  to parenting risk assessment services
    175–176
  from primary mental health workers 76,
    78, 81, 93
  and prioritisation 25–26, 91, 92
  re-referrals 95
  and sectorisation 93
  for self-harm 126
  and service development 25–26
  and specialist teams 94
  from Tier 1: 75–77, 79, 82–83, 162
  from Tier 2: 99
  and training requirements 94
  urgency 93, 110

Registered Mental Nurses (RMNs) 43
reviews of service provision 23
risk management 25

school nurses 78–79, 86
schools 85–86, 87
sectorisation 93
self-harm see deliberate self-harm
sensory impairment 105–106
serious mental illness 120, 121
service development plans 25–26
service users see user participation
social services departments, liaison with
  87
social workers 44, 87
special educational needs 86, 118, 137
special schools 137, 139, 140
staff rooms 5
staff support 24
staff training see training
standard setting and benchmarking 24
stigmatisation 79, 83, 84
strategic framework 9
strategy development 10
structure 3–4, 16–20
substance misuse 101
  and in-patient care 119, 123, 171–172
  and offending 179, 181, 182
  services see drug and alcohol teams
suicide 126, 129, 167, 180, 181
supervision 97
systemic approaches 2–3

teachers 85–86, 89
team working see multi-disciplinary
  working
Tier 1 professionals 1–2, 12, 17
  and autistic spectrum disorders 147
  and bereavement services 162, 165
  and challenges 80–81, 82–84
  and child protection 32
  guidelines and protocols for 79, 89
  and initiatives in Tier 1 working
    78–79
  liaison and consultation with see under
    liaison and consultation
  referrals 75–77
  and strategies for moving into Tier 1
    75–81
  support for 22, 25, 76, 77
  training for 64, 78–79
Tier 2: 12, 17
  and assessment 96
  and child protection 32
  and continuum of care 97
  'critical mass' of staff 96
  requisites of a service 96–97
  and supervision 97
  and training 97
  and treatment options 99, 100

Tier 3 teams 12, 17, 24
   and attentional problems services 150
   and autistic spectrum disorders services
      146–147
   CAMHS learning disability teams
      134–135
   and child protection 33
   and day patient services 112, 113
   and eating disorders 124
   and multi-disciplinary working 38, 95
   and paediatric liaison 109
   and referrals 94, 95
   and sensory impairment 106
Tier 4 link workers 124
Tier 4 services 12–13, 17
   centres of specialist forensic expertise 184
   and child protection 33
   and integration of tiers 4
   and management team 19
   and sensory impairment 106
   see also in-patient psychiatric care
tiered system 3–4, 12–13, 17, 18
Together We Stand 1, 9, 78
training 61–65
   of administrative staff 18
   and autistic spectrum disorders services
      147–148
   and bereavement services 164
   CAMHS as providers 64
   and clinical governance 22, 26
   and court work 73–74
   educational strategy 62
   and family therapy 102, 104
   and in-patient psychiatric care 122, 125
   inter-agency team training 63–64
   learning climate and methods of 62–64
   and learning disabilities services 140
   links with further education
      establishments 65

multi-disciplinary 63
   and referrals 94
   on self-harm management 130
   of teachers 89
   for Tier 1 workers 64, 78–79
   for Tier 2: 97
treatment interventions
   and court reports 67
   and evidence-based practice 51–52
   structuring and management of options
      96–106
trusts 20

user participation 2, 55–60
   active and passive involvement 55–56
   aims 56
   and clinical governance 23, 26
   documentation and management 59–60
   empowerment and ownership of process
      59
   ensuring diversity 58–59
   and learning disabilities services
      140–141
   participatory appraisal 56–58
   and synergistic interests 59
   and Tier 1 work 77, 80
   and Tier 2 work 99
   and whole community approach
      56–57

voluntary sector 2, 57

waiting lists 3, 25, 91
Welfare Checklist 28
welfare of child as paramount 27, 30, 31,
   54, 66

young offenders 67, 69, 178–184
youth offending teams 170, 180